Copyright

All rights reserved. This book or any portion thereof may not be used in any manner whatsoever without the express permission of the author.

Dedication

I am grateful to God for the gift of life. This book is dedicated to my wife, Jacqueline, and our kids Richie, Stanley, and Nana.

I am eternally grateful to my parents Mr. Stanley Norman and Mrs. Amma Akomaa Norman.

I would also like to use this to honour the memory of my in-laws, Mr Eddie Senah and Ama Adoma.

Table of contents

Chapter 1 6
    Introduction 6

Chapter 2 11
    The Best Healthcare systems in the western world 11

Chapter 3 15
    History of the UK's NHS 15

Chapter 4 18
    Structure of the NHS 18

Chapter 5 20
    Challenges faced by the NHS 20
        Funding 20
        Ageing Population 21
        Long waiting times 22
        Information Technology (IT) system challenges 24

Chapter 6 27
    Global demand for health professionals 27
    Health worker shortages across the developed world 29
        USA 30
        UK 32
        Canada 37

Chapter 7	38
Bureaucracy	38
Chapter 8	42
Money spent on locum/temporary staff	42
Chapter 9	43
Competitiveness of Salaries of UK Doctors	43
Chapter 10	45
Public health	45
Chapter 11	49
Eliminating waste	49
Chapter 12	50
Some Government interventions	50
The NHS Long-Term Plan 2019	50
NHS workforce plan	53
Chapter 13	55
Health financing	55
UK	55
Norway	60
Australia	62
The United States of America	65
Chapter 14	71

- Prescriptions for the NHS 71
  - Back to Basics 71
  - Financing the NHS 73
  - Money alone is not enough to address the NHS' problems......75
  - What COVID has taught us 76
  - Addressing staff shortages 81
  - Efficiency and cutting waste 85
- Conclusion 87
- References 90

Chapter 1
Introduction

I am a Ghanaian-trained doctor who worked in Ghana for almost ten years before joining the National Health Service (NHS) in the United Kingdom (UK). I spent most of my working time in the rural areas of Ghana and eventually rose to the level of a Senior Physician Specialist.

I have worked in the private and public sectors in Ghana and did previously run my own health facilities in Ghana. Improvement in healthcare delivery is a passion of mine.

I have worked across various roles since 2017 in my hospital in England. I initially spent a few weeks as a foundation year doctor (newly qualified doctor) before working as a medical registrar (training to be a consultant). I have also worked as a Specialty doctor, acting consultant in Geriatrics and then as a Specialist in Geriatrics. This has allowed me to see how the NHS works from a clinician's point of view across various levels of clinical work. I have also undertaken courses that have deepened my understanding of how the NHS works.

I have only worked in one district hospital in England and have not worked in any of the different countries of the UK. However, the issues are the same in the other countries of the UK. I have addressed this limitation by doing a lot of research on the various topics and referencing them. This book brings a lot of evidence-based discussions to the various topics.

My experience working in NHS England has been largely positive. This has been a good opportunity as Ghana's Health Service is largely modelled after the UK's NHS with the goal of achieving free health care at the point of need.

In 1948, the NHS became the first health system that offered free healthcare at the point of need (1). It performed the first liver transplant in Europe as well as the world's first Computed Tomography (CT) scan and In-vitro fertilisation (IVF) (1). The NHS celebrated its diamond anniversary on the 5th of July 2023 (1).

The NHS is one of the social interventions revered the most by the British people and is always one of the key topics during an election (2).

The UK NHS is the fifth biggest employer in the world employing 1.7 million workers in the UK (3). The UK NHS also sees a million patients every 36 hours (4).

The only UK government expenditure above that of the NHS is welfare (5).

A survey by two prominent UK think thanks, the King's Fund and Nuffield Trust, looked at the British public's sentiments towards the NHS (6). There is public goodwill towards the UK NHS with 62% of respondents in that survey saying the NHS made them most proud to be British (6).

The survey also showed most British people want the NHS to be accessible and free (6). Ninety-four per cent (94%) of British respondents agree that healthcare should be free whilst 84% want healthcare to be available to everyone (6).

I remember having a conversation with a colleague who told me some patient stories that highlighted all the positive sides of the NHS and some of the challenges it faces.

They did a life-saving intervention on a patient, which an audit showed would have cost hundreds of thousands of pounds.

Amazingly, this patient had this life-saving intervention and walked out of an NHS trust without paying a dime.

He also told the story of a British citizen living in the United States of America (USA) who relocated to the UK because he needed a huge amount of money for a medical procedure there. He moved to the UK to have this procedure at no cost whatsoever. Medical tourism is one of the challenges the UK NHS faces as people can access healthcare without paying the due tax.

These everyday stories and experiences are what endear the NHS to people in the UK.

I have taken advantage of my NHS experience to study a health system that was arguably the best in the world (7, 8).

However, the NHS has faced several challenges in recent years (9, 10). Accessibility is becoming a challenge and several years of underfunding has shaken the foundations of the NHS (10). Some of the areas that need to improve are health outcomes, cancer care and mental health provision (10). The coronavirus 2019 (COVID) pandemic placed further strain on the NHS.

I wrote a book in 2022 titled 'A developing country's Health System Challenges, addressing Ghana's No Bed Syndrome' (11). This book was largely a reflection of my previous experiences across Ghana and the UK vis-a-vis best practices in healthcare provision (11).

This book sought to address Ghana's health system challenges and proffer solutions to the aged long 'No Bed Syndrome' in Ghana (11). I would define the 'no bed syndrome' as the lack of an appropriately resourced hospital bed staffed by an appropriately skilled health worker (11).

I came up with these eight issues as the main challenges faced by Ghana's health sector (11):

1. Health financing

2. Structure of the health management system

3. Healthcare infrastructure and Information Technology

4. Human resource development

5. Emergency systems

6. Public health focus on disease prevention and community care

7. Public pride and goodwill toward Ghana's National Health Insurance Authority

8. Patient empowerment

Having worked in the UK for the past seven years, these same issues are faced by the UK and other developed countries. The only difference is the magnitude of the problems and the nature of the solutions required.

The UK also faces an ageing population with its attendant healthcare requirements (12).

Why have I felt the need to write this book? There is a saying in my language that the one who weeds the path does not always see that it is crooked. To wit, observers sometimes see wrongs which are not obvious to those involved in an activity.

I believe my 'few years' in the NHS and my outside experience mean I see things from a different lens. An example of this is a quality improvement project I did at the Harrogate District Hospital on medical registrar bleep numbers, which were outrageously high when

I started to work there. This was hitherto the norm. This quality improvement project contributed towards the use of the Ascom mobile device and the single point of access as referral tools for acute medicine admissions. This has improved the acute medicine referral processes in the hospital.

There is a need for NHS workers, who are on the ground, to share their experiences and find their voice in the debate about a fit-to-purpose NHS. Politicians alone should not shape the narrative.

The most important thing the NHS needs to do is to work more efficiently and for NHS workers and the public to design and implement locally grown solutions that would facilitate this.

The future NHS should be patient-focused, efficient, provide a great working environment and free at the point of care.

Chapter 2
The Best Healthcare systems in the western world

The Commonwealth Fund, an American health think tank, has been ranking healthcare systems in eleven developed countries every three years (7, 8).

The countries assessed are Australia, Canada, France, Germany, the Netherlands, New Zealand, Norway, Sweden, Switzerland, the United Kingdom, and the United States (US) (7, 8). Though it is difficult to compare health systems due to different environments, their ranking provides an objective assessment using key matrices (7, 8). They assessed **access** to healthcare, **administrative efficiency**, **equity**, **care processes** and **health outcomes** (7).

They used data from various bodies including the Commonwealth Fund international surveys, the Organisation for Economic Co-operation and Development (OECD) and the World Health Organization (WHO) (7, 8).

In 2017, the UK's healthcare system came up on top despite spending less on healthcare compared to some of the other countries. This was the second time in a row that the UK had topped this ranking (7).

Australia, the Netherlands, New Zealand, Norway, Switzerland, Sweden, Germany, Canada, and France followed in that order (7).

The US came last despite spending the most on healthcare provision (7, 8). The US spent 16.6% of its gross domestic product (GDP) on healthcare delivery (7, 8). The UK spent 9.9% of its GDP on health in 2019 whereas Australia spent 9% of its GDP in 2017 (8).

UK health expenditure as a percentage of GDP increased during the coronavirus-2019 (COVID) pandemic (9).

According to the Commonwealth Fund, the NHS did well on safety of care, the systems in place to prevent ill health, such as vaccinations and screening, and the speed at which people get help (7, 8). The UK NHS also did well with respect to equitable access to healthcare irrespective of income (7, 8).

The worst performance by the NHS was in health outcomes (7, 8). Compared to the other developed countries, the UK had poorer cancer survival rates with higher early deaths and poor general health of the population (7, 8).

The ranking

1. UK

2. Australia

3. Netherlands

4. New Zealand

5. Norway

6. Sweden

7. Switzerland

8. Germany

9. Canada

10. France

11. US

However, the UK's health system had fallen down the pecking order in the Commonwealth Fund's 2021 ranking (10). Now ranked fourth according to the think tank, Norway, Netherlands, and Australia ranked higher (10).

There was a dip in the UK's performance on health access, health outcomes and mental health provision (10). Mental health provision was a new parameter introduced by the think tank in 2021 (10).

The Washington-based Commonwealth Fund blamed this on a dip in access to healthcare as well as a lack of investment in the health service (10).

The UK NHS scored lower marks in 2021 compared with 2017 on three of the five domains: access to care; care processes, and equity (10).

"For example, nearly 60% of adults in the UK found it somewhat or very difficult to obtain after-hours care, one of the highest rates among the countries surveyed," Eric Schneider, the lead author of the Commonwealth Fund's 2021 report, said (10).

Again, while 78% of Britons in 2017 said that their regular doctor always or often answered a query on the day they posed it, there was a 12% drop in 2021 (10).

In addition, there was a 5% drop in the number of patients who saw a doctor or nurse on the same or next day the last time they sought care. This had dropped from 57% to 52% (10).

Furthermore, just 33% of patients said that they got counselling or treatment for mental health problems when they sought help from a specialist (10). The UK's health sector was the second worst performer of the eleven countries on mental health provision (10). Only France scored lower (10).

The UK ranked fourth for access to care, administrative efficiency, and equity, and fifth for care processes (10). Again, the UK NHS was just ninth for health care outcomes (10).

Despite a drop in the ranking, the UK NHS is still amongst the best healthcare systems in the world (10).

Siva Anandaciva, the chief analyst at the King's Fund, the leading UK health think tank has acknowledged delays in accessing healthcare in the UK (10). There were teething problems even before the coronavirus-2019 pandemic (COVID) (10). The UK had issues with a growing waiting list, inadequate funding, and a workforce crisis (10). Unfortunately, COVID has exacerbated these problems (10).

He also acknowledged the increasing demand for hospital, mental health and General Practitioner (GP) services across the UK health system (10).

Chapter 3
History of the UK's NHS

The UK realised the need to spend more on healthcare during World War 2 (13). In 1942, William Beveridge, a civil servant proposed a free national health service to tackle the country's problems (13).

The foundational basis for the NHS was to employ the British people and to use it to educate the people and to tackle disease (13).

The NHS Act was part of a social welfare policy under Clement Atlee's Labour government (13). This came at the right time as the UK was facing issues with food supply, a housing crisis, a severe winter, and spiralling tuberculosis (13).

The National Health Service Act passed by the new labour government in 1946 drew on previous experiences of an earlier, local version of the NHS in Wales in the 1930s (13).

There was opposition to the formation of the NHS (13). The British Medical Association (BMA) feared loss of income for doctors employed by the NHS whilst many local authorities and voluntary bodies feared the loss of control over the hospitals they run (13).

Others, including even Winston Churchill thought the NHS would cost too much to run (13).

Despite the opposition, the National Health Service was born on the 5th of July 1948 using taxes as a primary source of funds and aiming to provide free healthcare to all at the point of need (13).

The NHS brought many positive changes to Britain's health system (13). Amongst these were:

1. Free medical treatment for all British citizens.

2. The nationalisation of hospitals under the Ministry of Health and the formation of regional health authorities.

3. The creation of health centres to provide services like vaccinations, maternity care, district nurses etc.

4. A better distribution of doctors around the country with GPs, opticians, and dentists in every area (13).

'On 5 July we start together, the new National Health Service. It has not had an altogether trouble-free gestation. There have been understandable anxieties, inevitable in so great and novel an undertaking. Nor will there be overnight any miraculous removal of our more serious shortages of nurses and others and modern re-planned buildings and equipment. But the sooner we start, the sooner we can try to see these things and secure the improvements we all want. My job is to give you all the facilities, resources and help I can, and then to leave you alone as professional men and women to use your skills and judgement without hindrance. Let us try to develop that partnership from now on.'- Aneurin Bevan, The Lancet, 1948 (13).

At its inception, the National Health Service had 480,000 hospital beds in England and Wales with an estimated 125,000 nurses and 5,000 consultants (13).

Britain spent £248 million on the NHS in the first year, overspending by more than £140m (13).

Strict educational rules were relaxed in order to recruit more nurses to fill the gap of 48,000 in 1948 (13). As a result, the NHS had 245,000 whole-time equivalent nurses by 1952 (13).

Some of the successes of the NHS over the years are (14):

1. Healthcare has become accessible to all residents of the UK.

2. Life expectancy in the UK has increased.

3. Child and maternal mortality have come down.

4. Its involvement in major medical breakthroughs such as transplant surgery, cancer care etc.

5. Its involvement in disease prevention and screening services.

6. It helped in the provision of social care services (14).

Chapter 4
Structure of the NHS

The initial NHS structure comprised regional hospital boards that managed some hospitals, primary care providers who were contractors and not paid salaries by the government and community services (15).

Though there are some differences between the health management structures in the various countries of the UK, they are generally similar (15). The individual countries run their own healthcare system with funds provided by the central government (15).

The structure of the Health Service in England has changed over the years and comprises these bodies at present (15):

1. Secretary of State for Health and Social Care is the political head of the Department of Health and Social Care (15).

2. The Department of Health, which is responsible for government funding and policies (15).

3. NHS England, which is an independent body that oversees healthcare in England. NHS England merged with NHS improvement in 2019 but they have different boards (15).

4. Integrated care systems (ICS) that seek to integrate health care provision. They are replacing Sustainability and Transformation Partnerships (STPs) that brought together NHS providers, commissioners, local authorities, and other partners to serve the long-term needs of the local populations. STPs covered areas with populations of one to three million people (15).

5. Clinical commissioning groups (CCG) are a group of hospitals and services that provide NHS services within a catchment area (15).

Integrated Care Boards (ICBs) have replaced CCGs following further restructuring in 2022 (15).

6. NHS Foundation Trusts provide direct patient care after commissioning (15).

7. General practitioners (GPs) who provide some primary care services. GPs in England have formed primary care networks that cover a population of 30,000-50,000 people. This brings together GPs and local providers (15).

8. Secondary Care provides specialist emergency and non-emergency hospital care (15).

9. Tertiary care provides sub-specialist services (15).

10. The National Institute of Health and Care Excellence (NICE) provides standardised guidance on managing various conditions (15).

11. The Care Quality Commission (CQC) monitors health facilities and ensures patient safety and quality health provision (15).

12. Health Education England is the body that ensures the training of NHS workers (15).

The restructuring of the NHS in 2022 gave more power to the Secretary of State for Health and Social Care (15).

Chapter 5
Challenges faced by the NHS
Funding

Funding has been an issue from the onset, and this continues to put pressure on NHS budgets (16). Lack of funds has contributed to the growing waiting list for many operations and other services (16).

Increasing life expectancy and an ageing population continue to put pressure on the NHS (16).

The UK NHS is no longer completely free as it was at its inception since services such as eye tests and dental treatment are charged (16). Prescription charges were introduced only four years after its inception (16). However, free prescriptions were re-introduced in Wales in 2007 (16).

An article in the British Medical Journal (BMJ) outlined some of the challenges facing the NHS (16). It called for more commitment to social care reforms and funding as well as an effort to address health inequalities (16).

It also called for a closer integration of the NHS and social care, along with greater alignment of entitlements to health and social care (16).

It also advised more funding to match the current challenges and to improve future outcomes (16).

The article highlighted the need for a proper workforce strategy, revisiting priorities set out in the 2019 NHS long-term plan and considering the effects of the COVID pandemic (16).

It also highlighted the need for a stronger focus on prevention and a revamp of the depleted public health system (16).

The article also emphasized the need for greater collaboration between all stakeholders to develop homegrown solutions without great influence from Whitehall (16).

Ageing Population

The UK has an ageing population (17). This is due to increasing life expectancy and declining mortality rates (17). However, increases in life expectancy in the UK have stalled since 2011 (17).

The UK has nearly 12 million people aged 65 and above (17) with one in five people in the UK (21.8%) projected to be 65 years and over by 2030 (17).

The additional increase in the over-65-year population would be equivalent to the size of London in fifty years (17). Five million four hundred thousand (5.4 million) people out of this number would be 75 years and above with 1.6 million being over 85 years (17).

The over 85-year group is the fastest growing and is set to double to 3.2 million by mid-2041 and constitute 7% of the UK population by 2066 (17).

Furthermore, over 579,776 people are over 90 years whilst 14,430 are centenarians (17). The number of centenarians living in the UK has increased by 85% in the past 15 years alone (17) with an anticipated population of 21,000 by 2030 (17).

Male and Female babies born in the UK in 2018 are projected to have a life expectancy of 79.9 years and 83.4 years respectively (17). It is estimated that 23.4% of male and 29.2% of female babies born in 2018 will survive to the age of 100 (17).

Despite this, life expectancy in the UK is lower than in other developed countries (17). The UK's average annual life expectancy improvement was lower than the EU average for both men and women between 2011 and 2016 (17).

Increasing non-communicable disease burden as well as health and care system challenges have been proposed as possible causes (17).

Long waiting times

The NHS published an elective recovery plan in February 2022 (18) to tackle the problem of waiting lists. The goals were to increase NHS elective activity to 30% above pre-pandemic levels by 2024-25 and reduce two-year and one-and-a-half year waits by 2022 and 2023 respectively (19). It also planned to reduce waiting times for diagnostic tests, cancer referrals and outpatient appointments (18, 19).

One way the NHS sought to reduce the waiting list was through advice and guidance services, which allowed GPs to ask Consultants for advice before hospital referrals (19). The data showed an increase in these requests from 42,700 in January 2019 to 114,000 in December 2022, a 167% increase (19).

There have been varied results since the recovery plan was published (19). According to the NHS Constitution for England, 92% of patients should wait no longer than 18 weeks from referral to treatment (19). NHS figures show that this target was met in just over half of cases in December 2022, falling from 60.1% the previous month (19).

However, the target to eliminate two-year waits had been largely met by July 2022 with the numbers falling by 93.9% in 2022 (19).

NHS Providers Chief Executive, Sir Julian Hartley, commented: 'Trust leaders and their staff have made significant progress in reducing long waits for patients, which is remarkable given the challenging circumstances in which they're operating. Their success in virtually eliminating two-year waits for elective care and being on track to bring down 18-month waits by April is a testament to the hard work of front-line teams' (19).

Unfortunately, the ambition to eliminate 1.5-2 year waits by April 2023 was not met as the numbers grew from 45,200 to 48,500 between January and September 2022 (19). The more than one-year wait also grew from 300,000 people in February to 410,000 by November 2022 (19). The overall number on the waiting list had grown to 7.2 million by November 2022 (19).

Those waiting for more than a year to receive treatment was a mere 1,845 in February 2020, and according to the Institute for Fiscal Studies (IFS), "illustrates the broader challenge: while waiting lists are continuing to grow overall, it is not mathematically possible for the NHS to reduce the number of people waiting for all periods" (19). "Instead, it can only prioritise reducing some groups, such as those waiting more than two years, while other parts of the waiting list continue to grow" (19).

The Deputy Chief Executive of NHS Providers acknowledged that 'waits of 18 months or more had gone up, and trust leaders were deeply concerned that other pressures – including staff shortages and escalating strikes – could not only obstruct future gains but derail ones already made' (19).

Tim Gardner, Senior Policy Fellow at the Health Foundation, acknowledged that these are not just numbers but that there was real patient suffering behind the scenes (19).

An analysis by the IFS has shown that waiting time targets by the NHS would be missed (19). Waiting times are expected to flatten in 2023 and eventually decline in 2024 (19). The failure to meet waiting time targets has been attributed to the effects of COVID and other pressures on the health system (19).

The IFS analysis shows that the NHS treated 6.6 per cent fewer patients from the waiting list in 2022 than in the same period in 2019 (19).

The IFS postulates that overall elective activity levels will need to increase by 20.9 per cent in order to meet waiting list targets by 2024-25 even after accounting for the increase in guidance and advice services (19).

At current treatment levels, the NHS would need to increase treatment volumes by 10.3 per cent annually between February 2023 and March 2025 to achieve 97% of 2019 levels (19). This 10.3% is unlikely to be met considering treatment volumes grew by an average of 2.9 per cent annually between February 2015 and February 2020 (19).

I continue to meet an increasing number of people who are returning to their home countries for healthcare due to long waiting lists. Unfortunately, the private healthcare sector is not a viable alternative either, as it is not that advanced. Even those who have sought private care here are not having their needs met.

Information Technology (IT) system challenges

Guy's and St Thomas', one of the biggest NHS hospital trusts in the UK, was shut down for ten days due to IT failure (20). This is a patient safety issue as many healthcare providers are transitioning into paperless or electronic records (20).

IT infrastructure includes computers, servers, and networks, as well as the supporting processes and staff (20).

IT failures affect everything from accessing patient records, seeing allergies, checking blood tests or scans, or even prescribing life-saving treatment (20). Such failures also increase costs (20).

Unfortunately, the NHS has not prioritised investments in IT infrastructure and there have been attempts in the past to cut costs in that sector (20).

A recent survey of NHS trusts commissioned by NHS England shows that unreliable and slow IT systems do not improve user experience in using electronic health records (20). Unfortunately, clinicians, who use these IT systems daily, have not contributed to improving these systems (20).

The British Medical Association (BMA) estimates that 27% of NHS clinicians lose over 4 hours a week due to inefficient IT systems (20). Many healthcare personnel have experienced these inefficient IT systems (20).

My own experiences are that a lot of time is wasted when using various inefficient IT systems to access patient records. I recently recorded how much time I spent on the computer accessing patient records in comparison to the time spent directly seeing patients. I spent 75% of my time on the ward on the computer.

This is an inefficient use of my time. It also distracts clinicians from their primary work, which is to see patients. It, therefore, takes longer to see patients. This means more clinicians and nurses are required to see a smaller number of patients.

I am surprised that different NHS hospitals and providers use different IT systems. NHS workers who change jobs must learn how to use different IT systems. This is costly in terms of wasted time.

Again, the lack of integration of the NHS IT systems means it takes time to get patient records from various facilities. There have been countless times that we could not access the health records of patients because they were seen in different hospitals or health facilities.

This comes at a cost to the NHS as some investigations and examinations are repeated.

Chapter 6
Global demand for health professionals

Figure 1. Number of Doctors, Nurses, and Midwives per 10 million Population, 2011 (21).

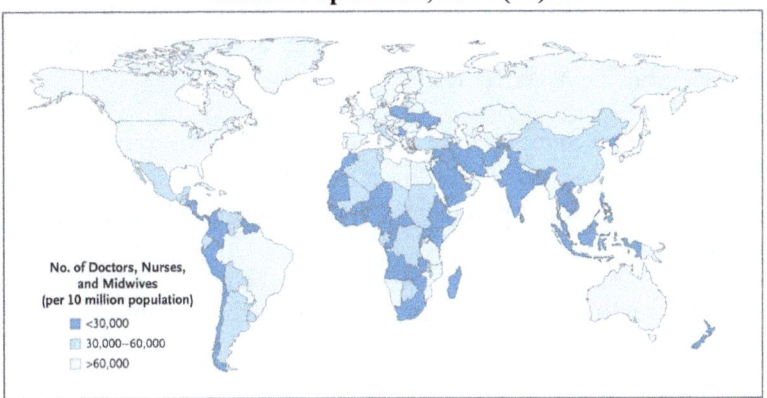

Data is from the World Health Organization (WHO) Global Health Workforce Statistics (21).

There is a shortfall of approximately 4.3 million doctors and nurses globally and this is particularly problematic in developing countries (21). Some fifty-seven poor countries have inadequate healthcare professionals, and this situation is exacerbated by the disease burden (21). The US is expected to have a shortage of 85,000 doctors by 2020 and 260,000 nurses by 2025 (21).

Demographic changes, epidemiology shifts, and redistribution of the disability burden have contributed to the need for more healthcare professionals (21).

The 2010 WHO Global Code of Practice has highlighted the need for richer countries to stop recruiting from poorer nations (22). As a result, the WHO has a red list of nations where direct recruitment of health workers by developed nations should not take place (22). The loophole that allows individual health workers to directly apply to work in developed nations has been abused (22).

Thirty-seven out of the fifty-five countries on the red list are from Africa with eight from the Western Pacific region, six from the Eastern Mediterranean region, three from the South-East Asia region and one from the Americas (23).

These red-listed countries have a Universal Health Coverage (UHC) Service Coverage Index that is lower than 50 and a density of doctors, nurses and midwives that is below the global median (48.6 per 10,000 population) (23).

All nations need to invest in their health and human resource needs (21).

The growing global demand for health workers has led to competition for health workers (21). Fast-growing countries, such as India, China, Brazil, and South Africa, even need more health workers (21).

Health worker shortages across the developed world

Germany

Germany has some 50,000 nursing vacancies at present (24). The German Nursing Council (DPR) predicts up to 300,000 nursing vacancies will need to be filled by 2030 (24). Germany also has an ageing population like most developed nations (25).

The German government launched a recruitment drive encouraging foreign nurses and caregivers to relocate to Germany (24). In 2019, the German health minister held discussions with Kosovo and Mexico on a recruitment deal (24).

Learning the German language and bureaucracy are some of the hurdles to the success of this recruitment drive (24).

A special agency to deal with immigration hurdles for foreign nurses and caregivers has also been formed (24). In 2020, 1,300 nurses from Mexico and the Philippines were waiting to have their applications processed in Germany (24).

Germany's drive for migrant workers contrasts with the move to restrict migration in other developed nations (25).

Germany has put in place a points-based system that factors in the migrant's age, skills, qualifications, and any link to Germany (25). They also plan to lower the salary, educational and German language requirements (25). Other incentives include migrant workers being able to bring families including their parents (25).

Migrants who meet the criteria can even move to Germany without a job offer (25).

USA

A study by Mercer shows the United States of America (USA) would have significant health worker shortages by 2026 with over 6.5 million of the 9.7 million healthcare workers in 2021 expected to leave in the future (26).

This would lead to a shortage of 500,000 employees in all states (26). There would be a shortage of more than 400,000 home health aides and 29,400 nurse practitioners by 2025 (26).

Concerns about health worker shortages had been raised at a 2019 US National Academy of Sciences workshop years before the Mercer study (27).

Americans are living longer, and an American Association of Medical Colleges (AAMC) report shows the over-65-year population will increase by 48% by 2032 (28).

The ageing population has exacerbated these health worker shortages, as older people require more medical care, often from Physician specialists, Geriatricians, and other specialists (29).

With many physicians due to retire, the American Association of Medical Colleges predicts a shortage of as many as 122,000 physicians by 2032 (28). The hardest hit areas would be the rural areas as they have fewer doctors (28).

Rural American states such as Utah, Vermont, and Tennessee, as well as remote territories like Guam and the Northern Mariana Islands, have the highest shortages of medical professionals per capita (26).

Though primary physicians including internists see the most patients, US doctors are choosing to specialise rather than enter primary care as these specialised fields are better recognised and remunerated (26).

Nurse and midwife Shortage in the US

According to the American Bureau of Labour Statistics, nurses especially degree nurses would be in high demand within the next decade (30).

According to the American Association of Colleges of Nursing (AACN), the US will need more than 200,000 new nurses each year until 2026 (31). This number is needed to fill new positions and replace retiring nurses (31). The USA also has a shortage of midwives (32).

Unfortunately, the US does not even have enough nurse educators to train the required numbers (30).

UK

There were 110,000 job vacancies across NHS trusts and many thousands more in primary care as of 2022 (33). There were 9217 advertised medical (and dentistry) vacancies for full-time equivalent jobs in NHS England alone in September 2018 (34). The specialties most affected are psychiatry, general practice, and emergency medicine (34).

The UK, with 2.8 doctors per 1000 population, has one of the lowest doctor-population ratios in Europe (34). The European average is 3.4 doctors per 1,000 population. Only four countries in Europe have lower numbers per capita than the UK (34). These countries are Ireland, Slovenia, Romania, and Poland (34).

Medical school places in the UK

The Royal College of Physicians issued a report in 2016 that said, 'the UK did not currently train enough doctors to meet demand' (34). Fewer people are also attending medical school (34).

A plan by the previous health secretary to achieve an additional 5000 GP posts by 2020 was not achieved (34). There were several contributory factors including low medical school numbers, poor retention of doctors and early retirement by doctors (34).

Medical school intake has been declining since 2010 from a high of 7500 in the late 1990s and early 2000s to only 5880 admissions in 2015-2016 (34).

The UK government plans to tackle this by expanding capacity at existing medical schools and building new medical schools (34). New medical schools in Sunderland, Lincoln, Angela Ruskin, Edge Hill, and Kent are expected to add an additional one thousand five hundred students (34).

The British Medical Association (BMA) raised concerns that it would take a decade before these plans translate to changes on the ground (34).

BMA medical students committee co-chair Harrison Carter affirmed the need to prioritise the retention of staff, as increasing medical school places alone would not address the shortfall (34).

Health Education England (HEE) estimates that England needs to train 8000 doctors a year to be self-sufficient. This gap has been filled by foreign trained doctors but 'the supply is drying up' (34).

Retaining doctors

Just over 30% of doctors are entering specialty training after their foundational training, according to a recent BMJ article (34).

Only 37.7% of trainees immediately took up a specialty training post upon completion of their training in 2018 compared to 42.6% in 2017 (34).

A General Medical Council (GMC) and British Medical Association (BMA) survey showed that burnout was a particular stumbling block to retention of doctors with 14.4% of doctors planning to take a career break (34).

A study of 12 cohorts of 30,272 doctors graduating between 1974 and 2012 in the UK found that 15% of the most recently qualified cohort were far more likely to report that they would probably leave the UK (34).

In 2016, the GMC issued 4,805 certificates of good standing to doctors considering leaving the UK (34). An increasing number of senior doctors are retiring early too with 721 GPs claiming their NHS pension on voluntary grounds in 2017, up from 198 in 2007 (34).

This has a part to do with large tax bills associated with pensions (34). A BMA survey in 2018 showed that more than half of consultants intend to retire at or before 60 years and half were less likely to take on extra work (34).

The chief executive of NHS Employers, Danny Mortimer has acknowledged the challenge of retaining senior clinicians (34).

The government has increased the maximum amount that retirees over 55 years who have accessed their private pensions can put in their pension from £4000 to £10,000 (35). The annual tax-free pension allowance has also been increased from £40,000 to £60,000 each year (35).

These changes mean less pension tax bills for doctors (35). However, the BMA has said it does not address all the issues especially those affected by the tapered annual allowance that has not been meaningfully reformed (35).

How many NHS staff are foreign nationals?

Around 220,000 out of 1.4 million NHS staff are non-British (36). This amounts to one in six NHS staff with a known nationality (36). As of 2022, there were over 200 nationalities working in the NHS with 7.2% being Asians and 5.3% from the European Union (E.U) (36). Thirty-one out of every 1000 NHS staff are African, and this number is growing (36).

Thirty-seven per cent (37%) of doctors working in the UK qualified abroad with over half obtaining their medical degrees in Asia (36).

Effect of BREXIT

Doctors from the E.U comprised 9.7% of the UK doctor population in 2018 (37).

A BMA survey of 1720 E.U doctors showed that 45% were considering leaving the UK because of BREXIT (37).

The Nuffield Trust evaluated the impact of Brexit on the UK workforce by focusing on four specialties: anaesthetics, paediatrics, cardio-thoracic surgery, and psychiatry (37).

These specialties were chosen as they have ongoing recruitment and retention issues and have a higher number of staff from the E.U and the European Free Trade Association (EFTA) countries (37). They looked at the increase in specialist or senior doctor numbers in these specialties in the five years before and after the 2016 EU referendum (37).

The survey showed a slowing down of the projected increase with nursing being particularly affected, increasing by only 29,000 (37). However, with 2010-2015 growth rates, this number was expected to be 87,000 (37).

Anaesthetics is one of the largest and most important specialties especially when it comes to surgical interventions (37). It has the highest number of E.U or EFTA doctors in the UK and faces significant workforce shortages (37). Using pre-referendum rates of increase, there should have been 2357 anaesthetists instead of the 1957 anaesthetists recorded in 2021 (37).

Cardio-thoracic surgery is another field that had many European doctors and where numbers have stagnated (37). There were 291 EU/EFTA cardio-thoracic surgeons in 2014 as against 268 UK-trained surgeons (37). This number has plateaued, and it is estimated that the UK would have had over 700 Specialists from the EU/EFTA region at previous rates (37).

Using previous growth rates, there would have been 288 more paediatric specialists and 165 psychiatrist specialists in the UK (37).

There would have been an extra 4000 specialists in the UK in 2021 alone using previous growth figures (37).

The uncertainty surrounding BREXIT seemed to be the reason for a slowdown in E.U/EFTA recruitment (37).

Industrial action by health professionals

Various health professionals across the UK have embarked on industrial action since 2022 thereby putting more strain on the NHS (38). This has largely been due to demands for better pay amidst the cost-of-living crisis in the UK (38). They have also suggested better pay would lead to better recruitment and retention.

The walkout by nurses and ambulance workers was the worst in the 75 years of the NHS (38). Physiotherapists have also walked out (38). The strike action by junior doctors in April 2023 led to the cancellation of 195,000 patient appointments (38). Twenty-seven thousand, three hundred and sixty-one (27,361) staff were absent from work at the peak of that industrial action (38).

There were 175,000 cancelled patient appointments in the junior doctor strike in March 2023 (39).

Canada

Canada ranked 26th out of 28 developed countries in 2016 when the physician-to-population ratio was analysed (40). Over six percent (6.6%) of Canadians reported they were unable to find a family physician in 2010 (40).

Despite Canada being amongst some of the highest spenders on health, she is ranked amongst countries with long waiting lists, low digitisation and a shortage of health professionals (40).

Canada's physician shortage is expected to be worse in the next ten years with recruitment of foreign-trained doctors being the only short-term solution (40).

Chapter 7
Bureaucracy

Figure 2: Picture of Dr Gordon Caldwell with all the forms needed for one medical admission

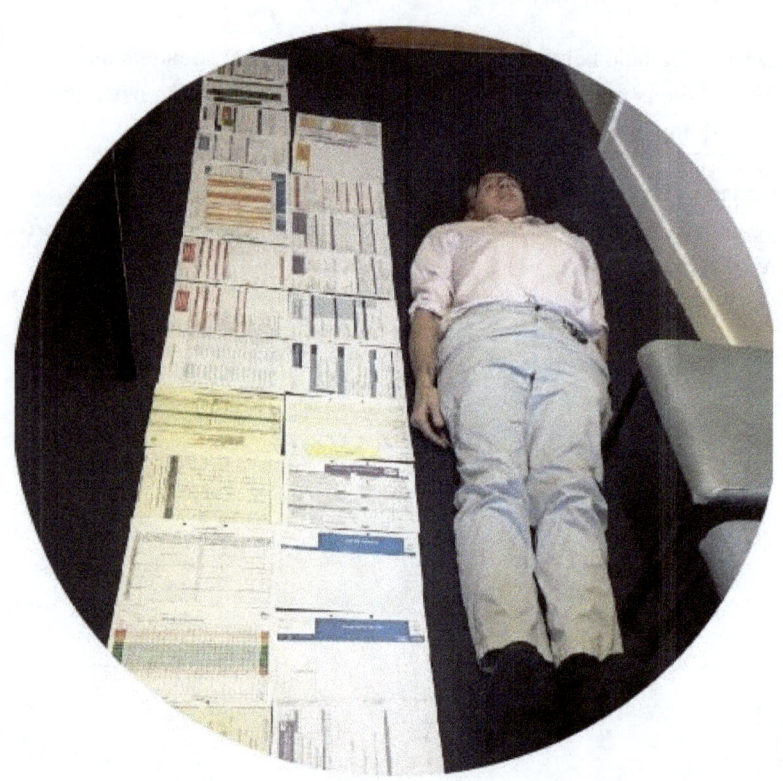

The Cambridge Dictionary defines Bureaucracy 'as a system for controlling or managing a country, company or organisation that is operated by a large number of officials employed to follow rules carefully' (41).

Bureaucracy has some advantages in healthcare as it is designed to manage risks including ensuring patient safety (42). However, excess bureaucracy affects efficiency and wastes the time of health professionals (42). This further affects staff performance and morale and can be counter-productive (42).

The UK spends less on administration compared to other European countries (7, 8). For instance, the UK spends a third less on administration compared to the Organisation for Economic Co-operation and Development (OECD) average and under half of that spent by Germany and France (7, 42). Expenditure on healthcare administration in the UK accounts for around 2% of healthcare expenditure (42) with non-clinical managers accounting for only 3% of the health service staff numbers (42). Managerial numbers have increased by only 1% in the decade up to September 2019 whereas the doctors and nurse population has risen by almost 10% (42). This indicates relatively high levels of efficiency (42).

While the UK's health system is more efficient when compared to the health systems in other developed countries, (7, 8) there is still room for improvement.

Clinicians are spending more time on administrative and other non-clinical mandatory requirements (42). For example, a community-based clinician spends about 30% of his or her time on administration and patient coordination (42). Additional mandatory work activities including appraisals have imposed more paperwork thereby taking more valuable time off clinicians (42).

The NHS Confederation is a membership organisation that supports partnerships and collaboration between various parts of the health and care system in the UK (42). It has called for more efficient processes that improve the quality and safety of healthcare provision and safeguards the time of health professionals (42).

'We have 152 versions of every wheel that's ever created. 152 contracts for purchasing home care services, adults safeguarding policies and procedures'. UK Home Care Association (42).

Examples of excessive bureaucracy are:

1) Duplicative data requests

2) Overly complex regulation

3) Lengthy appraisals and repetitive mandatory training

4) Time-consuming staff processes and information management

5) Out-of-date and overly prescriptive legislation

6) Time-consuming procurement processes (42).

As pointed out by Dr Gordon Caldwell in Figure 2, one must fill in so many forms as part of daily NHS work (42). Unfortunately, most of these have become tick-box events without contributing meaningfully to patient safety.

As he reiterated, these forms have been transferred to inefficient computer systems that often waste more time.

I have noticed the creation of too many job positions with some of these roles doing similar and overlapping things. This sometimes blurs the work and results in inefficiency. For instance, our hospital has the Supported Discharge Service (SDS) or Acute Response and rehabilitation in the Community and Hospital (ARCH) team, Urgent Community Response (UCR) team, hospital at home and virtual ward teams. All these are community teams involved in admission avoidance and early discharge services with overlapping functions and drawing on staff already in the system to provide these. These create shortages elsewhere as a result.

There are many jobs set up under various names, for instance under frailty or continence where already employed staff can and should perform said functions.

There are also many training requirements before NHS workers can perform procedures. I have seen several nurses who are better at putting in cannulae than some doctors, for instance. However, extensive training requirements means these nurses, especially the foreign-trained nurses, cannot help with procedures. Unfortunately, they would lose these skills with time.

Chapter 8
Money spent on locum/temporary staff

According to the NHS financial watchdog, NHS hospitals in England used to spend about half a billion pounds on private agencies to fill temporary vacancies (43).

NHS improvement data showed that some agencies charged £480 an hour for one Consultant with some trusts spending more than £2 million on the five highest-paid "locum" staff doctors in 2017 (43). Some of these locum doctors and nurses have been working at some hospital trusts for years (43). Caps on locum spending has reduced hospital expenditure by up to a third (43).

I am seeing an increasing number of junior doctors doing locum due to better remuneration and flexibility in working.

Hospitals are being encouraged to use bank staff to mop up extra shifts as this leads to about 20% in savings (43).

The NHS spent less on agencies in 2017 for the first time, saving £528m as a result (43). Fewer health professionals joined agencies due to more flexible working options and improvements in IT rostering systems (43).

These gains in 2017 have been eroded though with one NHS trust spending as much as £2500 for a single agency nurse shift in 2021-22 (44). The amount of money paid to agencies increased from £2.4 billion in 2020 to £3 billion in 2021-22, a 20% jump (44). Furthermore, NHS trusts in England spent £6 billion on bank staff in 2021-22 (44).

Chapter 9
Competitiveness of Salaries of UK Doctors

It takes many years at great expense to train a doctor and doctors are compensated for this by being some of the best paid professionals (45). UK doctors are outside the top 15 countries in terms of salary (45).

Data released by the UK student loans company in 2022 showed that a fresh doctor graduated with an average debt of £32,435 (46). The highest student loan was £121,400 (46). The average nursing student debt was £32,033 with the highest at £110,863 (46).

Tuition fees in public medical schools in the US range from $34,592 to $58,668 for residents and non-residents respectively (47). It costs $55,534 in private medical schools for residents and $56,862 for non-residents (47). Seventy three percent (73%) of newly qualified doctors in America graduate with a debt of $180,000 to $200,000 (47).

These are the rankings of countries according to physician salaries.

1. United States -Though the salaries of doctors in the US vary depending on location and specialty, the annual mean salary of a doctor in the United States is $294,000 (45).

2. Canada - The average salary of doctors in Canada is $278,000 per year (45).

3. Switzerland - Switzerland has one of the best healthcare systems in the world. Whilst a doctor in Switzerland earns on average $275,124 per year, some specialists can earn $746,030 per year (45).

4. Luxembourg - Doctors in Luxembourg earn on average $253,000 per year (45).

5. The Netherlands - General practitioners earn on average $117,000 whilst specialists earn around $253,000 per year (45).

6. Norway - Doctors in Norway earn around $196,834 per year (45).

7. Denmark - Doctors earn about $ 195,741 per year (45).

8. Finland - The average salary of doctors in Finland is $175,674 per year (45).

9. Belgium - Doctors on average earn $171,183 per year (45).

10. Germany - The average annual salary for a doctor in Germany is $166,000 (45).

11. Austria - Austrian doctors earn an average of $163,677 per year (45).

12. Australia - The average salary of Australian doctors is $156,000 per year with a starting salary of $129,188. The most experienced earn up to $234,000 annually (45).

13. France - Doctors earn an average of $130,361 per year (45).

14. New Zealand - The average annual salary is $105,828 with some earning up to $ 415,271 annually (45).

15. Ireland - Doctors on average earn $101,591 per year (45).

Chapter 10
Public health

Public health is "the science and art of preventing disease, prolonging life and promoting health through the organised efforts and informed choices of society, organisations, communities and individuals" (48).

The coronavirus-19 pandemic exposed weaknesses in the UK's public health system (49). According to data from John Hopkins University, the UK had recorded 24,658,705 COVID cases with 220,721 deaths as of October 2023 (49). The UK had one of the highest mortality rates in the world (49).

The troubles experienced by the UK during the COVID-19 pandemic have been blamed on inequality in the health system and the lack of public health experts (50). Only one trained public health physician was the chief medical officer at the beginning of the COVID pandemic (51).

I still remember my first experience of the UK's public health system when I had COVID. There were no contacts with me whatsoever apart from telling my employers. I felt lost in the system and there was no contact tracing.

The UK has the Scientific Advisory Group for Emergencies (SAGE) that provides independent scientific advice to the government (51).

People have suggested that there was political interference in the work of SAGE during the COVID-19 pandemic (51). For instance, the Prime minister's chief political adviser, Dominic Cummings and Ben Warner, his adviser on data science were present at several SAGE meetings (51).

This even led the UK's former chief scientific adviser, David King, to set up an alternative advisory group to provide the public with COVID-19 information (52).

There had been public health sector budget cuts of close to £1 billion prior to the COVID-19 pandemic (53, 54). There were budget cuts to local authorities too (53, 54).

The government published a COVID recovery plan with some structural changes to the public health sector (18).

There have been changes to Public Health England (PHE) because of the challenges encountered during COVID (55). The UK Health Security Agency (UKHSA) (55) has replaced Public Health England. This transferred Public Health England's health improvement functions to the Department of Health and Social Care, while its health protection elements form part of the new government agency (55).

The new public health authority, UKHSA, would prioritise the non-communicable disease burden by focusing on obesity, smoking, drug, and alcohol misuse, improving sexual and reproductive health, and promoting positive mental health (55). There would be up scaling of screening programmes and NHS health checks and improvement in mental health provision (55).

There would be a renewed focus on health security and health improvement (55). Health security focuses on protecting the population from infectious diseases and external health threats (55). The new public health department, which came into fruition in 2021, would give impetus to these functions by allowing greater cooperation and autonomy (55). It also aims to improve the use of relevant technology and prepare the UK for future pandemics (55).

The UK Health Security Agency will also combine PHE and NHS test and trace (55). Furthermore, national disease registry functions will also move to NHS Digital (55). A new office for health promotion has been set up to promote good health across the UK (55).

A white paper outlines the renewed focus on population health (55). These changes have been driven by lessons learned during the COVID-19 pandemic (55).

The new public health system calls for statutory integrated care systems and greater collaboration with local authorities (55). To ensure the independence of public health advice to the government, the Chief Medical Officer (CMO) would become the lead independent public health advisor (55).

An article by Drs Emily Oliver and Nicholas Segaren called for more public health training for doctors (56). Public health is a well-established specialty training though not enough clinicians are going into the field (56). I know of only one doctor who intends to go into public health in all my seven years in the UK.

The article emphasized the need for clinicians to have a better understanding of public health in order to better understand the health needs of patients (56). They argue that clinician involvement in public health would lead to more research and improvement in clinical practice (56). Programme evaluation as a part of public health also helps clinicians determine the value of their services (56).

They also emphasized the need for doctors to be better trained in management and leadership with a particular focus on financial and organisational management skills (56). Getting clinicians involved in public health would improve efficiency and result in health reforms (57). This would lead to a bottom-up approach instead of a top-down approach to service reform.

Doctors are generally expected to be leaders in the health sector and champion changes that benefit patients (58). For instance, the Mid-Staffordshire inquiry showed that a lack of leadership could have adverse effects on patients (58).

The article emphasized the need for public health training right from medical school to the postgraduate level (56).

Chapter 11
Eliminating waste

In an article in the BBC, Nick Triggle asked readers to send questions on the NHS (59). What readers wanted to know was "How much of the NHS budget gets spent on administration, settling lawsuits, internal market; what's left for treatment? Is this poor value?" (59).

A hospital nurse mentioned filling out 37 forms to admit a patient and then going ahead to input more data electronically (59).

The article also mentioned that extensive documentation, which is meant to avoid medico-legal issues, wastes resources (59).

A recent government-commissioned review by Labour peer Lord Carter says the NHS could save £5 billion by cutting waste (59).

Areas identified for savings include better management of staff absence, efficient procurement practices, more efficient use of space (he found one trust that used only a third of its estate for care), greater use of cheaper generic medicines and efficient working by health professionals (59).

An estimated £2 billion a year was being wasted through unnecessary investigations and treatments (59).

A report by the Public Accounts Committee, for instance, showed that the UK Department of Health spent £12 billion on personal protective equipment (PPE) between 2020-21 (60). The Department of Health argued that it needed to buy PPEs at a high cost due to the competitive pricing at that time (60).

The UK government wrote off £8.7 billion worth of PPEs out of this amount (60). The Public Accounts Committee also found that some £4 billion worth of unused PPE did not meet NHS standards (60).

Chapter 12

Some Government interventions
The NHS Long-Term Plan 2019

In 2019, key stakeholders in the UK drew a ten-year plan to improve the NHS and make it more efficient (61). Extensive consultations and thousands of submissions went into the drafting of that document (61).

These were the goals of the 2019 NHS long-term plan (61).

Maternal and child morbidity and mortality

1. Half the stillbirths and maternal mortality.

2. Ensure women who would derive the most benefit from continuity of care get it during and after their pregnancy.

3. Tackle prematurity by providing extra support for expectant mothers.

4. Expand mental health support during the perinatal period.

5. Tackle childhood obesity.

6. Provide more funds for the mental health needs of children and young people.

7. Reduce waiting times for autism assessments.

8. Ensure children with a learning disability get the right care.

9. Deliver world-class care using technology.

10. Ensure children with cancer get the best care (61).

Non-communicable diseases (NCD)

1. Reduce the non-communicable disease burden by preventing 150,000 heart attacks, strokes, and dementia cases.

2. Public health focus on NCD prevention by focusing on education and exercise programmes.

3. Save 55,000 more lives a year by early diagnoses of cancer.

4. Early diagnoses and treatment of lung conditions.

5. Spend at least £2.3billion more a year on mental health provision and ensuring more people get treatment. Mental health provision would focus on depression, anxiety, and those with severe mental illness (61).

Support for the aged

1. Increase primary and community care funding by at least £4.5 billion with a focus on more care in people's homes.

2. Ensure better coordination of older people's care.

3. Better support for care home residents and carers.

4. Improve care for people with dementia.

5. Improve end-of-life care (61).

The NHS long-term plan also outlines how these goals would be achieved (61). This includes:

1. Integrated care systems (ICS): better collaboration between NHS organisations and partners to ensure people get more control over their health and the care they receive.

2. Public health focus on NCDs; particularly focusing on the most vulnerable communities and people.

3. Improving the attractiveness of the NHS by attracting and retaining staff. Also, aim to train more health professionals.

4. Using technology to better deliver patient care.

5. Working with NHS workers to find better ways of delivering care.

6. Reducing administrative and procurement costs (61).

Virtual ward plans

Virtual wards are wards created to deliver the same level of hospital care for appropriate patients in their own home or usual place of residence (62). They receive daily remote monitoring and treatment for a short period of up to 14 days (62). A Multi-Disciplinary Team (MDT) that includes a consultant practitioner or GP (62) monitors such patients daily. Virtual wards are IT heavy and allow remote monitoring of patients (62). It also uses the same means to communicate with patients and other team members. This provides an alternative to hospital admission and helps with earlier discharges (62).

The UK government hopes to tackle hospital congestion by treating 50,000 patients a month through virtual wards (63). This is an up-scale as some 10,000 patients were thought to have received care through virtual wards or hospital-at-home initiatives in December 2022 (63). This has been a result of learnings from COVID-19 management (64).

The government mentioned the provision of high technology-laden virtual wards towards the end of 2023. However, no additional investments were announced (63).

Virtual wards are being developed by many local councils to cater for a range of conditions including respiratory conditions, COVID-19, heart failure and acute frailty (63). Eighty-six percent (86%) of ICSs are already implementing or planning to implement technology-enabled virtual wards (63).

Acute respiratory conditions and acute frailty conditions account for about 50% of patients who are suitable for the hospital at home and virtual ward models of care (63).

NHS England and NHS Improvement (NHSEI) expected to achieve 40–50 virtual wards per 100,000 population by December 2023 (65).

According to an analysis done by NHSEI, efficient use of staff time to deliver 50 virtual beds is equivalent to 31 additional secondary care beds (65). NHS Staff who cannot physically see patients may also work in virtual wards (65).

There is a growing evidence base for virtual wards with positive feedback from patients and broad clinical support (63). The provision of timely MDT through virtual ward models has led to a reduction in ED visits and hospital admissions (63).

There is an overlap with hospitals at home, which may require in-person reviews as part of the monitoring and treatment (63).

NHS workforce plan

The UK government has drafted the first workforce plan that seeks long-term solutions to its workforce crisis (66). It aims to provide £2.4 billion over the next 5 years as part of a 15-year plan (66). The plan published in June 2023 emphasises recruitment and retention of staff and training more health professionals through apprenticeships (66).

It aims to:

1. Double medical school places to 15,000 a year.

2. Increase GP training places by 50%.

3. Double nurse and midwife training places to 24,000 a year.

4. Increase those trained through apprenticeships to one in five.

5. Ensure 2000 people are awarded medical degrees through apprenticeships.

6. Consult on cutting medical degree duration to four years.

7. Provide an extra 60,000 doctors.

8. Increase assistant roles like nurse associates five-fold.

9. Increase NHS workforce by 300,000 by 2036/7.

10. Expand dentistry-training places by 40%.

11. Use technology including Artificial Intelligence (AI) and robotics (66).

Chapter 13
Health financing
UK

Taxes and National Insurance (N.I) contributions are the main sources of health financing in the UK with about 99% of the UK's Department of Health's budget coming from taxes (67). Charges for dentists' and optician's services as well as for prescriptions account for the remaining (67).

The UK government planned to spend around £122 billion on health in England in the 2017/18 health budget, or roughly £2,200 per person (67). Around £108 billion of that amount was expected to be used for the daily running of the NHS (67). The remaining money is used for public health activities, education, training, and infrastructural development (67).

In the UK, health spending was expected to rise to £123 billion in the 2020/21 budget (67).

NHS Scotland, Wales, and Northern Ireland (Health and Social Care Service) are almost fully funded by the various governments (67). Health expenditure per capita in 2017/18 was £2,500 and £2,300 in Scotland and Wales respectively (67). It was £2,700 in Northern Ireland (67). There are no prescription charges in these countries (67).

The Health and Social Care Levy imposed an increment in National Insurance (N.I) contributions and this has been used to partly fund healthcare from 2023/24 (68).

Before this, cuts had been made to expenditure on buildings, equipment, training more staff and disease prevention (68).

Most publicly funded social care in England is means tested with those having assets worth £23,250 and more normally not eligible for residential care (69). Local authorities spend on social care though some get grants from the central government (69). The total amount spent by the UK government on adult social care in 2019/20 was £23.3 billion, which in inflationary terms was only £99 million more than in 2010/11 (69).

According to the National Audit Office, the British people spent £10.9 billion in 2016/17 on social care (68, 69).

Many people who receive publicly funded social care contribute to it and this stood at £3.1 billion in 2019/20. This figure has risen in each of the past four years (69).

NHS providers and commissioners were required to increase mental health funding and balance their books by 2023/24 (70). A review of this soon realised the need to scale back financial incentives and cancel the historical debts of commissioners and providers (70). The market-like mechanisms, which emphasized competitiveness, are being ditched with a focus on more collaborative work in line with the NHS long-term plan (70).

The new NHS five-year funding deal and ongoing clinically led review of access standards may lead to a balance between performance and funding (71). Funding was a problem even before COVID and there is a need to find a more sustainable means of funding the NHS (72).

RAND Europe was commissioned by the Health Foundation to research how various countries in Europe fund their healthcare (73). It also looked at funding options for the UK's NHS and social care and assessed their acceptability to the British public (73).

Their report showed that the British people had a poor understanding of how the NHS and social care is funded especially the large private funding of social care (73). The report showed nationwide support to provide additional funds for social care (73). The British people support a collective approach to raising additional funds for health and social care (73). They also preferred those with a higher income paying more but did not support any age group paying extra (73).

The British public would want a public body to raise any additional funds for the health and social care sector (73). There is also support for these funds to be solely used for the purposes for which they were raised (73).

These preferences cut across the British population once age and socio-economic characteristics are controlled (73).

Private spending by the NHS

Some people believe NHS spending in the private sector is underestimated (74). David Rowland, who has extensive experience in the NHS and affiliated bodies, disputes the often-quoted figure of 7% (74). The source of the 7% figure is depicted in table 1 (74).

Table 1: Departmental Expenditure Limit -Department of Health and Social Care.

Table 1: Expenditure on non-NHS bodies	2018-19	2017-18	2016-17	2015-16	2014-15	2013-14	Increase 2013/14 to 2018/19	% increase 2013/14 to 2018/19
Independent Sector Providers	9,180,000	8,765,000	9,007,000	8,818,000	8,067,000	6,467,000	2,713,000	42
Voluntary sector	1,619,000	1,564,000	757,000	545,000	526,000	510,000	1,109,000	217
Local Authorities	2,889,000	2,737,000	2,909,000	2,869,000	1,774,000	2,473,000	416,000	17
Devolved Administrations	50,000	43,000	73,000					N/A
Total Spend on all non-NHS bodies	13,749,000	13,109,000	12,746,000	12,232,000	10,367,000	9,450,000	4,299,000	45
Total RDEL	125,278,000	120,650,000	117,031,000	114,730,000	110,554,000	106,495,000	18,783,000	18
Spend on private sector as a % of RDEL	7.3	7.3	7.7	7.7	7.3	6.1		0
Spend on all non-NHS as a % of RDEL	11.0	10.9	10.9	10.7	9.4	8.9		0

Note: RDEL stands for Resource Departmental Expenditure Limit. The data is taken from departmental accounts and annual reports (75).

In his analysis of the 2013/14 and 2018/19 fiscal years, the amount of money spent by the NHS on private providers is higher if various expenditures are accounted for (74).

He argues that NHS expenditures such as those used to outsource care from independent providers for elective surgeries etc. were excluded from private care (74). He also argues that independent primary care providers such as pharmacies, dental, eye and GP practices were excluded from the funds for private care (74). In addition, many social care providers are independent providers but were omitted in the initial calculation (74). Furthermore, the 7% was calculated using the total amount given to the Department of Health and Social Care rather than that given to the NHS (74).

In his calculation, he included expenditures both by Clinical Commissioning Groups and NHS Trusts on the independent sector, local authorities and the voluntary sector, all expenditures on primary care services which are delivered by independent contractors, all expenditures by the NHS on social care and the total amount given to NHS England each year rather the total amount of funds available to the Department of Health and Social Care (74).

In 2018/19, £29 billion or 26% of total expenditure by NHS England was on the independent sector (74). This amount has remained largely the same for the past six years (74).

He posits that the amount spent by the NHS on sourcing private services is £21 billion or around 18% of total expenditure even if GPs are excluded (74).

He argues that the NHS spends more on the private sector than is generally accepted or known to the public (74).

Norway

Figure 3: Organogram of the Norwegian Health system (76)

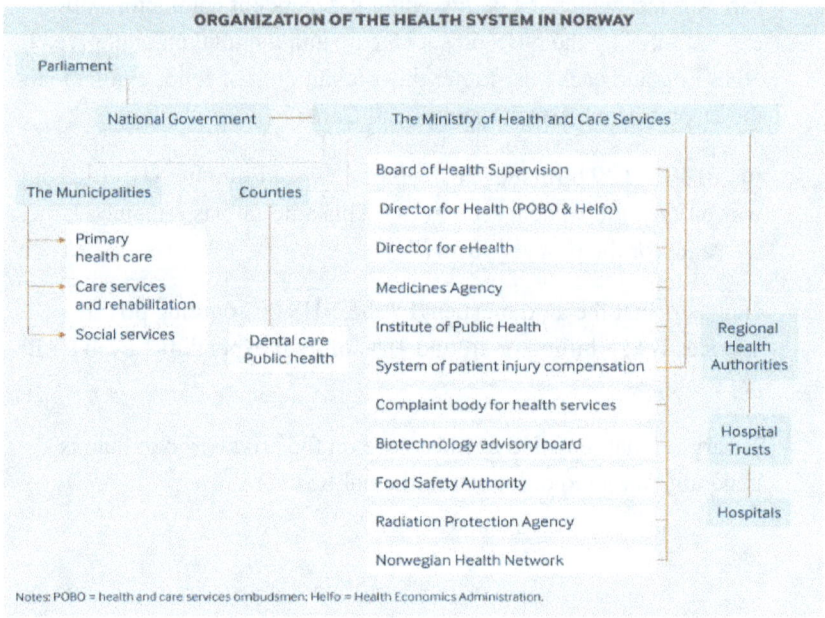

Norway provides automatic enrolment into a universal health coverage that encompasses primary, ambulatory, mental health, and hospital care, as well as select outpatient prescription drugs (77).

There is also co-payment with caps on how much one can pay (77). This health-financing model is funded by taxes and contributions from employees and employers (77). Public funds account for 85% of Norway's health expenditure. Norway spent 10.5 per cent of its 2016 GDP on health, an amount equivalent to NOK 68,065 (USD 6,647) per person (77).

Its health and social insurance coverage, known as the National Insurance Scheme (NIS), or Folketrygd is presently regulated by the 1997 National Insurance Act and the 1999 Patient Rights Act (77). There used to be an optional health insurance scheme in 1909, which covered employees and their families, but this was replaced by mandatory and universal health insurance in 1956 (77).

The Norwegian government regulates, funds, and oversees the provision of care (77). There is layered responsibility with municipalities in charge of primary care, preventive, long-term care and public health (77). The national government takes care of higher-level care through four Regional Health Authorities (RHAs) (77).

Ten per cent (10%) of Norwegians have private insurance that gives them the ability to choose providers and have quicker access to healthcare (77).

The Ministry of Health and Care Services provides political direction whereas the Directorate of Health implements health policies (77). The National Board of Health Supervision is the central supervisory body (77).

Residents need a Norwegian ID number to access healthcare (78).

Employers enroll their workers automatically and employees contribute through payroll (77).

Foreigners in Norway can access healthcare services through the Norwegian Health Economics Administration (Helfo) (78).

Australia

Australia's health system has multiple sources of funds (79). Funds are derived from all levels of government, non-government organisations, private health insurers and individuals who pay out-of-pocket costs for products and services that are not fully subsidised (79).

In 2016–17, the Australian government contributed only 41% of its nearly $181 billion on health with state and territory governments contributing 27% of the amount (79).

Australia spent 10% of its GDP on health in 2016-17 (79).

Australia's health system is a complex mix of service providers serving the Australian government, state and territory governments and the non-government sector (79).

The Australian government as well as state and territory governments are generally responsible for the running of their health system (79). The private for-profit and not-for-profit sectors also operate public and private health facilities in addition to providing private health insurance products (79). Australia's health workforce is similar to that of the UK, but they operate in a variety of health settings from large city hospitals to rural small clinics (79).

The Australian Government develops health policies, funds universal health insurance scheme, engages in health and medical research and provides funds to states and territories for public health services (79).

State and territory governments fund and manage public hospitals, deliver community public health services as well as regulate and license private hospitals (79).

Local governments in some jurisdictions are involved in providing public health services (79). All levels of government are also involved in the training of health professionals (79).

Medicare

Medicare, which is a universal health insurance scheme, is funded through taxes collected by the Australian government (81). Other means of funds include a Medicare Levy and a Medicare Levy Surcharge (79, 80) (Australian Taxation Office, 2021). Australians have free access to public hospitals and subsidised prescriptions (81).

Medicare is presently available to Australian and New Zealand citizens, permanent residents in Australia, and people from countries with reciprocal agreements, which includes the UK (Department of Health 2019) (81). Those without these entitlements must pay the full fees or buy private insurance (Private Health Insurance Ombudsman 2019) (79).

Private health insurance

Medicare does not usually cover ambulance services, optical aids, or most dental services (81, 82). This is usually covered by private insurance, which also confers the benefit of choosing one's doctor (82).

The Australian Government offers a means-tested rebate to people who hold private health insurance and surcharges higher-income earners who do not have a particular form of private health insurance (81).

The Australian government was expected to spend $105.8 billion on healthcare in the 2022-23 budget year (83). This was 16.8% of the government's total expenditure (83). However, this was expected to decrease by 4.4% up to 2026 due to the cessation of COVID-related payments (83).

Medicare and private health insurance rebate expenses would account for $39.5 billion, or 37.3% of total health expenses in 2022–23 (83).

Subsidies on medicines would account for $17.2 billion, or 16.3% of total health expenses in 2022–23 (83).

Funding to the states and territories will account for $27.3 billion or 25.8% of total health expenses in 2022–23 (excluding National Partnership payments) (83). There are also payments to veteran hospital services (83).

There are also expenses on public health, medical research, mental health provision, blood and blood products, other allied health services and health infrastructure (83). This accounted for 14.5% of total health expenses in 2022–23 (83).

Administration, health workforce investment measures and support for rural health initiatives was expected to cost $4.2 billion, or 4.0% of total health expenses in 2022–23 (83). However, this was expected to reduce by 22.5% between 2022–23 and 2025–26, largely due to the cessation of COVID-19 measures (83).

Aboriginal and Torres Strait Islander healthcare expenditure accounted for $1.1 billion or 1.1% of total health expenses in 2022–23 (83). Once again, this expense is expected to reduce due to the cessation of COVID-19 measures and other reasons (83).

The United States of America

Figure 4: Organogram of USA Health System

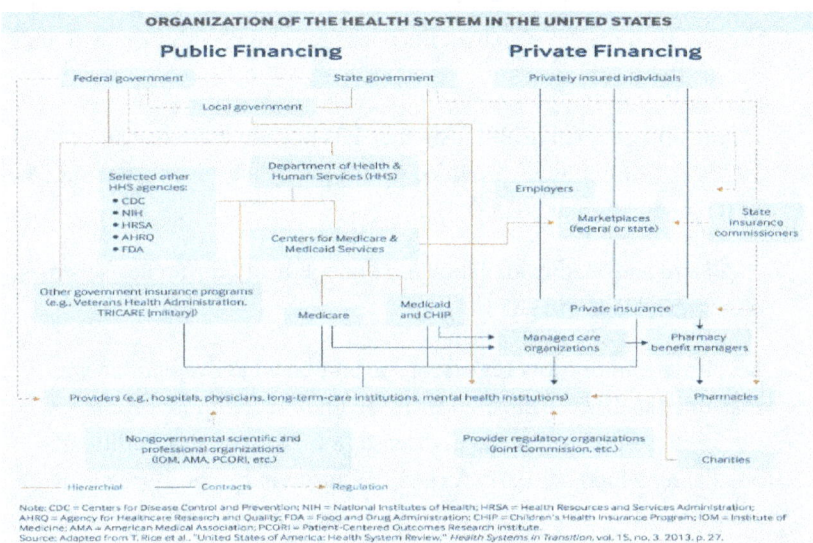

The United States (US) has multiple health insurance systems, with around one-tenth of the population uninsured (84). The US does not have universal health insurance coverage for its citizens (84).

Most Americans have private health insurance while two major federal government health insurance programmes, Medicare, and Medicaid, offer coverage for the vulnerable (84). The vulnerable include people with disabilities, the elderly, and the poor (84).

Out-of-pocket payments per capita for coinsurance, co-payments, and deductible amounts, have increased substantially in real terms in recent years (84). Even for those insured, high out-of-pocket costs are barriers to receiving timely care and treatment (84).

Public funding accounted for 45% of total healthcare spending in the US in 2018 (84).

States ensure local coverage of health insurance whereas public and private insurers agree on benefits packages and cost sharing with their clients (84).

Employer-provided health insurance has been in existence since the 1920s (84). Employers provided health insurance cover for about 55% of the population in 2018 (84).

Medicare and Medicaid, which are Federal health insurance schemes, were introduced in 1965 (84).

Medicare initially was for persons aged 65 and above but this was expanded in 1972 to encompass those under 65 with long-term disabilities or end-stage renal disease (84, 85). There is traditional Medicare, which has parts A (hospital insurance), and B (medical insurance) (84, 85). One can have coverage either through traditional Medicare or Medicare Advantage (Part C), under which people enroll in a private health maintenance organization (HMO) or managed care organization (84, 85). Part D allows a voluntary outpatient prescription drug coverage option to be provided through private providers (84, 85).

Part A, or hospital care, covers hospice and short-term skilled nursing facility care too (84, 85).

Medicare Part B covers physician services, durable medical equipment, home health services, short-term post-acute care such as rehabilitation services in skilled nursing facilities or in the home and very limited outpatient prescription, dental and vision services (84, 85).

Medicaid, which provides health insurance for 17.9% of Americans, provides coverage for the vulnerable including low-income families, people with disabilities and children up to 18 years (84, 86). Medicaid is means-tested and requires annual renewal (84, 86).

Medicaid covers a broad range of inpatient and outpatient services including long-term care, diagnostic services, family planning, maternity services, and transportation to medical appointments (84, 86).

The Children's Health Insurance Program (CHIP) was created in 1997 to care for those not eligible for Medicaid but cannot afford private insurance (84). Its use varies from state to state (84).

The Affordable Care Act (ACA) was passed in 2010 to increase access to health insurance in the US (87). It made it mandatory for most Americans to obtain coverage and expanded the coverage of the various health insurance schemes (87). This resulted in 20 million more people receiving health insurance coverage in the US (87).

The US government facilitated this by providing more funds and premium subsidies through legislation and regulating pharmaceutical products and medical devices (87).

The ACA required employers with 50 or fewer employees to cover 10 essential benefits (87). These included ambulatory care, emergency services, hospitalization, obstetrics, mental health services, prescription drugs, rehabilitative services and devices, laboratory services, preventive and wellness services, chronic disease management, paediatric services, dental and optician services (87).

Private health insurance

Federal taxes account for 63% of Medicaid funding whereas state revenue accounts for the rest (84, 86). The care of more than two-thirds of Medicaid beneficiaries is privately managed and paid through capitation (84,86).

Capitation is a provider payment system in which health providers are typically paid in advance at a pre-determined fixed rate to provide a defined set of services for each client for a fixed period. The providers are paid irrespective of any service provision during the designated period (88).

The fixed amount paid for a health capitation system is typically paid on a Per Member Per Month (PMPM) basis (88). Under the capitation health payment system, the member or subscriber selects a preferred primary provider (PPP) to provide all the services under the capitation basket in exchange for the capitation rate (88). The total capitation amount would then be transferred to the provider at the beginning of the service period with the calculated amount based on the total number of members who have selected a given provider (88).

Medicare on the other hand is funded through a mix of federal taxes, mandatory payroll tax for Part A and individual premiums (81, 84). In 2019, over 30% of Medicare beneficiaries decided to receive it through a private Medicare Advantage health plan (89).

One-third of total American health expenditure in 2018 was privately funded (90). Sixty seven percent (67%) of Americans have private insurance with employers sponsoring 55% of that and 11% privately purchased (90). Employer-sponsored insurance covers workers and their dependants but does not usually cover dental or optical services (90).

Individual Americans paid 10% of total health care costs out of pocket in 2018 (90). Households paid as much as the federal government for healthcare within that period (90). Individuals pay more for dental care (40% of total spending) and medications (14% of total spending) with the average payment by a single person being $1846 in 2018 (90).

Some private providers provide charity and uncompensated care to the non-insured (90). The non-insured can also access emergency care as guaranteed by law (90).

Primary care physicians, which includes specialists in family medicine, general practice, internal medicine, paediatrics, and some elderly care physicians, make up the chunk of all professionally active doctors (91).

Approximately half of primary care doctors owned their practices in 2018 with general internists owning more private practices than family practitioners (91) do.

Primary care physicians are paid through a combination of private and public insurance with 66% of their revenues coming from fee-for-service payments (92). Medicare and Medicaid have relatively lower reimbursement rates so not all specialists accept publicly insured patients (92, 93). Specialists who see outpatients are also free to choose the type of insurance they would accept (93).

Most specialists operate single-specialty group practices in both private practices and hospitals (93).

A few providers accept only cash due to the bottlenecks or delays associated with reimbursement of co-payments (93).

Though primary care physicians are not required to provide out-of-hours care, 45% provided out-of-hours care in 2019 (94). This is usually provided in private clinics and largely caters for younger, healthier individuals (94).

Both generalists and specialists provide mental health services with most patients seen in the outpatient department (95). The Federal Substance Abuse and Mental Health Services Administration provides grants to states for community mental health services (95).

Medicaid accounts for most long-term care needs whereas Medicare and most employer insurance plans cover only short-term post-acute care services (96). Private insurance for long-term needs is rare (96).

The ACA initially included the Community Living Assistance Services and Supports Act for long-term care, but this was repealed in 2013 as it was deemed unworkable (96).

Attempts to lower costs

The US has the highest Health expenditure per capita in the world at an average of $11,172 in 2018 (97). In addition, healthcare costs have grown between 4.2 per cent and 5.8 per cent annually over the past five years (97).

The Federal government attempts to controls costs by setting provider rates for Medicare and the Veterans Health Administration, use of capitation payments, capping out-of-pocket payments, requirements for private insurers to submit prospective rates for State or Federal review, use of lower cost formulary and through rebates (97).

Federal hospitals are also required to openly post and update costs of medical procedures annually (97).

Employers have also tried to eliminate agencies that act as intermediaries to lower costs (97). Some companies like Amazon, Berkshire Hathaway and JP Morgan have also teamed up to form their own non-profit healthcare corporations (97). Other companies also provide on-site health clinics (97).

Chapter 14
Prescriptions for the NHS
Back to Basics

Figure 5

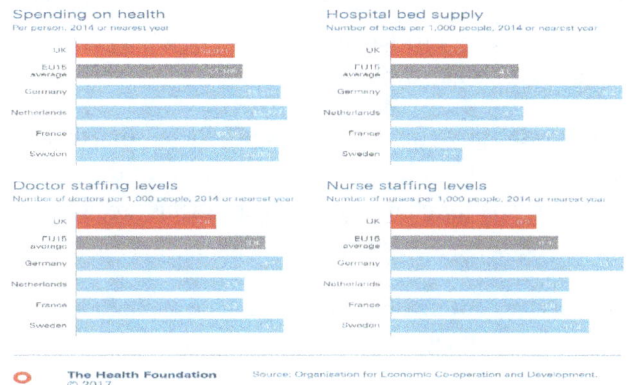

The UK needs to increase the number of hospital beds and the staff needed to manage these beds. I cannot see an alternative to this. Whereas there were 480,000 hospital beds in the NHS in 1948 (98), there are only 141,000 hospital beds today (99).

A very recent article in the medical journal Age and Ageing looked at the evidence behind the use of virtual wards (62).

It found that there was not a lot of data on virtual wards as compared to hospitals at home models (62). In addition, it could be potentially costlier as the costs to patients and families had not been factored in previous cost estimates (62). It concluded that research and evaluation should be an integral part of virtual ward models (62).

Virtual wards are supposed to use high-level IT systems to deliver virtual hospital-like care in people's usual residences.

My experience talking to clinicians involved in virtual wards showed that they had not yet received the required IT tools. A simple tool like an Electrocardiogram (ECG) was not even available to them.

In addition, members of our team were moved to cover this new 'virtual ward', which is largely a hospital at home. This means the same workforce was being juggled around creating shortages elsewhere. This creates a gap cycle.

Therefore, it seems the government has staked a lot on something, which has not proven to be efficient yet (62). Virtual ward team composition and criteria for choosing the right patients are not even clear (62).

I am surprised this was not implemented in an incremental manner before the nationwide rollout.

Financing the NHS

The elephant in the room is finding a sustainable NHS financing model. I have reviewed various financing models in some developed nations including that of the UK in earlier parts of this book. The sustainability of the NHS using the current funding sources has been questioned (71, 72) and a new and sustainable source of funding has been suggested.

I disagree with this view. I believe that the UK government can and is able to provide the necessary funds to the NHS as it has done with other priorities recently. However, the challenge is political will. Therefore, it is imperative that a new funding model takes this out of the hands of politicians.

A new financing model must also address new sources of funds and ensure increased and sustainable funding. Furthermore, any new funding option should be acceptable to the British public. Taxes are the main source of funding currently and increasing taxes or borrowing are funding options.

I propose a tweak of the current financing model to include a bit of the Norwegian model. The NHS can implement NHS numbers or cards, which everyone must have to access the NHS free of charge. A fee of 20-100 pounds can be charged per year based on the income received by UK residents. Those earning more would be expected to contribute more and employers can deduct this automatically. This is similar to the current financing model that utilizes National Insurance contributions to fund healthcare.

The survey on public sentiments about the NHS shows that people are willing to pay more for 'free' NHS services at the point of care. In addition, high-income people paying more for NHS services would be acceptable to the British public. This would subsidize costs for low-income earners and the vulnerable.

Using this model, the NHS can generate between £1.38 billion and £1.71 billion extra per year or per month (if this is charged monthly). This was calculated using a UK population of 68,979,510 as of 2023 (100) with an average of 6% of the population earning £50,000 and above (101).

We can incentivize people to pay this by giving a percentage of this contribution back as a pension if they use the NHS less. We can define what 'using the NHS less' means. It would also inspire people to be more proactive with their health since healthier people would use the NHS less. People would be self-motivated to cut down on excess alcohol, smoking and other unhealthy lifestyle habits. This idea would incorporate a tweak of the Singaporean model.

The 'vulnerable' can have free NHS numbers. A clear criterion for the 'vulnerable' would be needed.

The NHS numbers or cards would eliminate medical tourists getting healthcare free of charge, as one would need an NHS number or card to access healthcare. Medical tourists would be expected to pay for any care received under the NHS or, as I suspect, would choose to access private health care thus taking some work off the NHS.

Of course, anyone in an emergency should be able to access the NHS without paying anything immediately. They can be billed afterwards.

Money alone is not enough to address the NHS' problems

Berkshire Hathaway Inc. Vice Chairman Charlie Munger has criticised the US healthcare system for being expensive and inefficient (102).

He argued that the healthcare system in Singapore was more efficient though it costs 20% less than that of the US (102).

Despite the United States spending the most on healthcare per head than any other country, life expectancy is lower, and mortality is higher than in other developed countries (7, 8, and 84). Moreover, healthcare outcomes are low and mixed at best (7, 8). It has the highest level of treatable and avoidable death as well as maternal and infant mortality when compared to other developed nations (7, 8, and 84).

Despite the need for more spending on the NHS, just throwing money at the problem would not solve the problem. Moreover, its financial sustainability would be a challenge without making the NHS more efficient.

What COVID has taught us

COVID mortality was highest in Europe and the Americas with 10 out of the 20 countries with the highest mortality being in Europe (103). The US topped with the highest COVID mortality and morbidity (103).

On the contrary, ten countries with the lowest COVID death count per million were in Africa and Asia (104). There have been accusations that the UK made several mistakes in its handling of the COVID-19 pandemic. As a result, a public enquiry was set up (103).

Although it is difficult to compare countries based on their COVID response and outcomes, the developed world can learn some things from the developing world when it comes to public health (103).

The lower mortality and morbidity in Africa have been attributed to a younger population, different ways of recording death, greater use of outdoor spaces and potentially protective antibodies (103).

Despite this, others have highlighted the good work done by developing countries that drew on their experiences in managing infectious diseases (103). They responded earlier and forcefully and drew on their previous experience with Severe Acute Respiratory Syndrome (SARS), Middle East Respiratory Syndrome (MERS) and Ebola (103). I remember Ghana already required masks and testing at the airport whereas the UK had no such measures earlier on in the COVID pandemic.

Though the developed world was heavily hit by COVID, some countries like Germany and New Zealand were thought to have handled it well too (104).

Good leadership, learning from previous experiences and being innovative were some of the strengths of the developing world (104).

This is something even developed nations can learn from especially in a globe, which is increasingly connected (104).

Good leadership

African countries tried to contain and prevent the disease by acting decisively and quickly (104). Some closed their borders quickly (104). Mauritius for instance started airport screening for COVID and quarantining visitors from high-risk countries two months before its first case (104). Nigeria had a task force set up within 10 days of its first case (104). Contrast this with the UK whose first COVID case was on 31st January 2020, but an action plan was unveiled in early March (104).

Because of their experience with Ebola, African countries understood the need to work together (104). Africa had already set up the Centres for Disease Control and Prevention (CDC) (104). The African CDC, for instance, launched the Partnership to Accelerate COVID-19 Testing (PACT), which aimed to increase testing capacity and deploy better-trained health professionals in the various countries (105).

The African Union also established a continent-wide platform to procure laboratory and medical supplies (104). This allowed equitable sharing of resources compared to the competitive practices developed nations adopted (104).

They also called on captains of industries to help. Zimbabwean billionaire, Strive Masiyiwa, led private sector contribution (104). He leveraged technology and partnerships locally and abroad to do this (104). There are now plans to expand these to hospitals and local authorities across member states. These decisive actions paid dividends (104).

Though the European Union has a common platform called the Joint Procurement Agreement, slow bureaucratic processes meant some countries set up parallel structures (106).

The Vietnam government also showed strong leadership in its COVID fight and Vietnam had one of the lowest COVID mortalities (104). They were successful in getting the population involved in COVID mitigation measures (104). Akin to the African experience in containing Ebola, Vietnam had learnt lessons from the 2003 SARS outbreak (104). They designed effective containment measures including quarantine based on exposure risk rather than symptoms (104).

Uruguay, with one of the highest elderly populations in South America, also learnt from best practices by using aggressive COVID-19 testing and drawing on strong societal support (107).

Innovation

Senegal and Rwanda developed ways to lower COVID-19 testing costs (108). Senegal for instance developed a ten-minute COVID-19 test that costs less than US$1 whereas Rwanda scientists developed a way to pool many samples together to test at a go (108). They used the data to map disease burden and hot spots (108).

In Ghana, for instance, drones were used to disinfect open-air markets and other public spaces (109).

These cost-effective and improvised ways could be learnt by the developed world considering the economic burden of COVID (104, 110).

The spread of COVID from a small town in China, Wuhan, to the whole world has shown that governments across the world need to cooperate and learn from each other to address global health issues (111).

Developed nations also refused to share COVID-19 vaccines and technology with developing countries that are still under-vaccinated

(112). This was myopic in my view as the COVID pandemic clearly showed the interdependence of the global village.

The UK and other developed nations relied on technology instead of in-person contact tracing (104). This did not prove effective (104). The use of the COVID app in the UK had many challenges with a lack of public trust and ownership (104).

Developed nations are less inclined to learn lessons from the healthcare systems of the developing world, as there is a perception that the knowledge and expertise in developing countries are not relevant to the local circumstance of developed nations (104).

A rapid evidence review published by the Ada Lovelace Institute concluded that there was no evidence to support the effectiveness of digital contact tracing or immunity certification (113). The institute has called for the establishment of a new Group of Advisors on Technology in Emergencies (GATE) to oversee the development and testing of future digital tracing applications (113).

I remember the first two times I had COVID. There was no follow-up or contact by anyone apart from my hospital, which knew for work purposes. I completely felt lost in the system.

As in the 1918 Influenza pandemic, the COVID pandemic showed that the public health foundations of infection prevention, isolation or quarantine and even simple mask-wearing still work.

The Public health sector needs to be reformed. Public health training should be an integral part of medical training and we must encourage doctors to pursue this specialty.

Addressing staff shortages

The UK government's workforce plan (66) is a step in the right direction. It aims to recruit and retain health and social care staff through a long-term funded plan with emphasis on apprenticeships (66).

Many clinicians are burnt out because of the demands of their work (33) as they have to grapple with inefficient IT systems coupled with increasing demand from patients and relatives (33, 20).

Elsevier Health collaborated with market research company Ipsos to look at the expectations of clinicians of the future (114). The study involved three phases (114). The first phase was an hour's interview with 23 healthcare leaders from across the world to gauge expectations of future clinicians (114). The second phase was a 15-minute online global survey completed by 2,838 clinicians in 111 countries to gauge attitudes and discover possible solutions to the challenges faced by clinicians (114). The final phase comprised three round tables with key opinion leaders in the US, UK, and China to gather reactions to the findings and provide expert points of view on the clinician of the future (114).

Their findings show that more clinicians are burnt out and are considering leaving the profession (114). To address these challenges, clinicians are calling for more well-being support as well as more efficient technology in healthcare delivery (114).

Widespread workforce shortages in the UK have led to burnout amongst staff (33). For instance, managers at the Royal Preston Hospital in the UK have shared some employee sentiments (33).

"We have witnessed senior experienced staff crying with frustration and anger... [they are] mentally drained and despite their best efforts have seen patients suffer and have received negative comments from distraught relatives and carers" (33).

Though the COVID pandemic exacerbated these issues, there were teething problems before COVID.

Healthcare workers want more efficient working systems and IT. They also need more flexible working patterns that allow better work-life balance.

Despite the need for more health professionals including nurses and doctors, people interested in pursuing this pathway are not receiving the financial support they need.

A friend of mine who is a student nurse has struggled to pay her fees. Despite her commitment, she has not received the financial support needed. She tells me some nursing students have already dropped out of school as a result. The UK government should give financial incentives including supporting the fee payment of people who take up training in such fields.

This financial support should be repaid to the state if beneficiaries fail to complete their school or leave the NHS on completion. They should be expected to work in the NHS for a number of years on completion of their training.

Many people are unhappy about the role of Physician Assistants/Associates (PAs). They are worried this would dilute the work of doctors and that these PAs would not be able to provide the quality of care required. Furthermore, there are concerns they would take up the slots reserved for doctors who need supervision.

Ghana has been using PAs for a long time and some of these legitimate concerns have been raised there too. I worked with many PAs in different hospitals in Ghana. I was also involved in the training of PAs. I have witnessed a wide range in the clinical skills and knowledge of PAs. PAs even practice independently in some healthcare centres in Ghana and it is hard to distinguish between them and doctors sometimes. The Medical and Dental Council of Ghana, Ghana's version of the GMC, currently regulate PAs. Ghanaian PAs have asked for more and more rights as the years have passed.

The use of PAs is one way to bridge the clinician shortage in the UK. Advanced clinical practitioners already perform similar functions. Unfortunately, they are usually drawn from existing workers thereby creating a shortage elsewhere.

The use of PAs would fail to address the workforce challenges if the foundational problems are not addressed. We need to create an attractive working environment and make remuneration competitive.

There must be more emphasis on the regulation of PAs, and this is where I feel the British Medical Association must channel its resources. We must also anticipate future attempts to give even greater responsibility to PAs.

The NHS needs to employ more Specialty and Specialist doctors (SAS). Some of these are senior clinicians, usually foreign-trained and consultants in their own country but chose not to pursue the consultant training process in the UK. Some of these doctors are more experienced, senior, and better skilled than some of their UK consultant colleagues.

Remuneration for these roles must reflect the experience of the employees. The NHS should simplify the processes for highly skilled foreign-trained professionals to work as consultants or senior clinicians.

Those in the specialist position require a minimum of 12 years of medical or dental practice, of which a minimum of six years should have been in a relevant specialty. I propose that specialist doctors who have been in that role for five years are allowed to be on the specialist register as consultants. They are already performing all the roles expected of consultants. This will make the position more appealing to highly skilled clinicians worldwide. It would also address the senior clinician challenges and ensure there is high-level senior decision-making across the NHS.

Patients would benefit from having hospital-based doctors, as continuity of care would improve. Some SAS doctors also work in primary care and the community.

It would also save the NHS money as it costs over £500, 000 to train a consultant.

As SAS doctors do not need to rotate around, this offers stability to those already in those roles. This would be more attractive to clinicians with families. So, this alternative pathway to be a consultant would be more acceptable to those looking for a better work-life balance.

This aligns with the goals of future clinicians, according to recent studies.

Efficiency and cutting waste

Despite increasing numbers of health professionals and more money being pumped into the NHS, more needs to be done. The NHS needs to find efficient ways of working.

With a skeleton staff on the wards during recent NHS junior doctor's strikes, I was amazed we could do most of the work with less than half our usual staff numbers. Of course, those working were senior clinicians and therefore the quality and speed of decision-making was good and probably avoided delays.

There were more discharges in one of those strikes than there had ever been in the hospital. There were also fewer patient falls than usual. This showed how a more efficient system could work with a lower number of health professionals. However, senior clinicians cannot do overtime consistently.

Nurses need to work efficiently too. For instance, many patients on the wards can independently take their medications. In fact, they do so at home. However, the nurses habitually take over this responsibility, which sometimes results in delays to drug administration and complaints from patients. Allowing such patients to take their own medications would save the nurses some time, which they can use on other important tasks. There are mechanisms to do this. However, the processes to do this should not be so laborious that it is easier for the nurses to administer them.

We use various IT systems to access patient records, and this takes a lot of our time. I believe I spend more time with these IT systems than I do with patients on the wards. In addition, one sometimes cannot even access the health records of patients within the same region. I believe strongly that healthcare providers in the UK must use the same IT system and the government must invest in this as a matter of priority. The use of efficient technology for patient management is key.

I still remember the ridiculously high number of bleeps I would receive as a medical registrar on call in my early days in the UK. This was brought to the fore due to an audit or quality improvement project I did. This brought real changes to how acute medicine referrals were done. The use of the Ascom mobile device for routine referrals at the Harrogate District Hospital instead of pagers has made referrals more efficient.

Another area of waste is the use of consumables. As someone who worked in a developing country before working in the NHS, I cannot help but see the many times we throw away consumables because we have taken more than we need, or we realised we didn't need it. Or the many times we request blood tests the patient has just had or are unnecessary.

This place is where most NHS workers need to play a big part. We must immerse ourselves in quality improvement projects and audits that make our work better and more efficient. This is something that only we the workers on the ground can do. People often do tick-box quality improvement projects rather than embark on projects that would bring real positive changes on the ground.

There were 7.2 million missed GP appointments in England alone in 2019. This waste amounted to £216 million. It also costs about £42 to see a GP, £367 for an ambulance transfer to the emergency unit, £86 if someone receives the lowest care at the emergency unit, at least £418 if someone receives more complex treatment and investigations and £901 per day for long stays.

I believe people should pay the cost of missed NHS appointments, if there are no good reasons.

Conclusion

The UK NHS is still ranked high amongst the best healthcare systems in the world despite its many challenges (7, 8).

The Commonwealth Fund, a US think tank that ranks the healthcare systems across eleven developed nations has ranked the UK NHS fourth in its latest ranking, falling from its previous number one ranking (7, 8).

The UK NHS fell down the pecking order because of a lack of investment in its running. It had lower marks with respect to health access, equity, administrative efficiency, and care processes. The NHS also had poorer outcomes in terms of cancer treatment, health outcomes and mental health provision.

The NHS is facing several challenges, including inadequate financing, a workforce crisis, an ageing population, long waiting lists, and a lack of efficiency.

The global demand for health professionals means the NHS is competing for global talents. The government's workforce plan, which includes amongst others the plan to increase the number of apprenticeships and other clinical roles, would seek to improve staffing levels. Some of the ways to make the NHS attractive to global talents include paying competitive salaries and enhancing the conditions of service of healthcare workers.

According to revealed statistics, the NHS has spent over £1 billion remunerating doctors to pick shifts during the recent strikes by doctors. However, the BMA estimates £1 billion is needed to pay the salary increment they desire accounting for taxes that the government would get back. The government argues that £2 billion is needed. Again, the NHS spent £3 billion a year on agencies and an extra £6 billion on bank staff in 2021/22 (43, 44) It also spends on private institutions to try to clear the waiting list backlog. Though striking doctors and the government must come to a reasonable compromise, the government is surely paying that money in other ways.

The UK NHS also needs a sustainable funding source. A study to assess the British public's sentiments towards the NHS found that most people want the NHS to be free at the point of care. They also support more funding for the NHS and social care. They also support the idea of higher-income people paying more to support the health needs of the least paid and vulnerable (6, 73).

I have proposed an NHS number or card, which would be renewed annually or monthly at a fee based on income and funded by the British public. One would need this to access free healthcare in the UK. This would generate additional money that can be used directly by the NHS.

I propose that a portion of these contributions should be reimbursed upon retirement if the service is used less. Using the service less can be defined as a certain number of visits per year. This would also incentivize people to prioritise their health.

Research has shown that future health professionals are looking for a better work-life balance, more efficient ways of working and better support at work (114). I have therefore proposed another pathway to being a consultant that offers a better work-life balance.

Furthermore, doctors need to take up more leadership roles, especially in public health.

Though quality improvement is embedded in the NHS, NHS workers themselves must own this. The NHS needs to find more efficient ways of working and the workers on the ground would be key if this is to succeed. Research shows the NHS can save £5 billion annually if it cuts waste (59).

I believe my parent hospital has made the correct diagnosis by recommitting to quality improvement with a focus on patients.

Finally, money alone is not enough to address the NHS' problems. It needs to find more efficient ways of using its limited resources. This can be done through better use of technology and greater involvement of NHS workers and the public.

QR code for reviews

References

1. NHS England (2023). *NHS England» About the NHS Birthday*. [online] www.england.nhs.uk. Available at: https://www.england.nhs.uk/nhsbirthday/about-the-nhs-birthday/.

2. The Independent. (2019). *NHS overtakes Brexit as voters' top priority for election, poll finds*. [online] Available at: https://www.independent.co.uk/news/uk/politics/nhs-concerns-brexit-general-election-boris-johnson-corbyn-poll-a9211196.html [Accessed 6 Mar. 2024].

3. Alexander R. Which is the world's biggest employer? BBC News [Internet]. 2012 Mar 20; Available from: https://www.bbc.co.uk/news/magazine-17429786.

4. How much money does the NHS waste? (2016). *BBC News*. [online] 21 Oct. Available at: https://www.bbc.co.uk/news/health-37715399.

5. Statista. (n.d.). *Benefit expenditure in the UK 2020*. [online] Available at: https://www.statista.com/statistics/283954/benefit-expenditure-in-the-uk/.

6. Wellings, D. (2022). *Has the public fallen out of love with the NHS?* [online] The King's Fund. Available at: https://www.kingsfund.org.uk/blog/2022/10/has-public-fallen-out-love-nhs.

7. Triggle, N. (2017). NHS ranked 'number one' health system. *BBC News*. [online] 14 Jul. Available at: https://www.bbc.co.uk/news/health-40608253.

8. Gulland, A. (2017). UK has best health system in developed world, US analysis concludes. *BMJ*, [online] p.j3442. doi:https://doi.org/10.1136/bmj.j3442.

9. Prendergast, T. (2022). *Healthcare expenditure, UK Health Accounts - Office for National Statistics*. [online] www.ons.gov.uk. Available at: https://www.ons.gov.uk/peoplepopulationandcommunity/healthandsocialcare/healthcaresystem/bulletins/ukhealthaccounts/2020.

10. Campbell, D. (2021). *NHS drops from first to fourth among rich countries' healthcare systems*. [online] the Guardian. Available at: https://www.theguardian.com/society/2021/aug/04/nhs-drops-from-first-to-fourth-among-rich-countries-healthcare-systems.

11. Norman D. A developing country's health system challenges; addressing Ghana's 'no bed syndrome'. Available at: https://www.amazon.co.uk/developing-countrys-health-system-challenges-ebook/dp/B09SY772JC.

12. www.ons.gov.uk. (n.d.). *National population projections: 2018-based - Office for National Statistics*. [online] Available at: https://www.ons.gov.uk/releases/nationalpopulationprojections2018based.

13. Tweddell, L. (2008). *The Birth of the NHS – July 5th 1948 | Nursing Times*. [online] Nursing Times. Available at: https://www.nursingtimes.net/archive/the-birth-of-the-nhs-july-5th-1948-08-01-2008/.

14. www.longtermplan.nhs.uk. (n.d.). *NHS Long Term Plan» The NHS in England at 75: priorities for the future*. [online] Available at: https://www.longtermplan.nhs.uk/publication/the-nhs-in-england-at-75-priorities-for-the-future/ [Accessed 6 Mar. 2024].

15. Paul (n.d.). *Structure of The NHS - The Medic Portal.* [online] www.themedicportal.com. Available at: https://www.themedicportal.com/application-guide/the-nhs/structure-of-the-nhs/?v=79cba118546 [Accessed 6 Mar. 2024].

16. Ham, C. (2020). The Challenges Facing the NHS in England in 2021. *BMJ*, [online] 371(371), p.m4973. doi: https://doi.org/10.1136/bmj.m4973.

17. Raleigh, V. (2022). *What is happening to life expectancy in England?* [online] The King's Fund. Available at: https://www.kingsfund.org.uk/publications/whats-happening-life-expectancy-england.

18. NHS England (2022). *NHS England» NHS publishes electives recovery plan to boost capacity and give power to patients.* [online] www.england.nhs.uk. Available at: https://www.england.nhs.uk/2022/02/nhs-publishes-electives-recovery-plan-to-boost-capacity-and-give-power-to-patients/.

19. Blaazer, G. (2023). *NHS waiting times unlikely to fall in 2023: IFS.* [online] Hospital Times. Available at: https://www.hospitaltimes.co.uk/nhs-waiting-lists-unlikely-fall-2023-ifs/.

20. Zhang, J., Budhdeo, S. and Ashrafian, H. (2022). Failing IT infrastructure is undermining safe healthcare in the NHS. *BMJ*, [online] 379, p.e073166. doi:https://doi.org/10.1136/bmj-2022-073166.

21. Crisp, N. and Chen, L. (2014). Global Supply of Health Professionals. *New England Journal of Medicine*, 370(10), pp.950–957. doi:https://doi.org/10.1056/nejmra1111610.

22. www.nhsemployers.org. (n.d.). *Code of Practice red and amber list of countries | NHS Employers*. [online] Available at: https://www.nhsemployers.org/articles/code-practice-red-and-amber-list-countries.

23. WHO renews alert on safeguards for health worker recruitment [Internet]. www.who.int. Available from: https://www.who.int/news/item/14-03-2023-who-renews-alert-on-safeguards-for-health-worker-recruitment.

24. Welle (www.dw.com) D. Germany looks abroad for nurses, caregivers | DW | 14.08.2020 [Internet]. DW.COM. Available from: https://www.dw.com/en/germany-looks-abroad-for-nurses-caregivers/a-54576126.

25. Germany passes law to attract skilled migrant workers amid fierce debate. BBC News [Internet]. 2023 Jun 23; Available from: https://www.bbc.co.uk/news/world-europe-66003238

26. Major US Healthcare Labor Shortages Projected in Every State by 2026, Mental Health Professionals Grow in High Demand, Mercer Report Shows [Internet]. www.businesswire.com. 2021. Available from: https://www.businesswire.com/news/home/20210929005680/en/Major-US-Healthcare-Labor-Shortages-Projected-in-Every-State-by-2026-Mental-Health-Professionals-Grow-in-High-Demand-Mercer-Report-Shows

27. Institute of Medicine (US) National Cancer Policy Forum. Supply and Demand in the Health Care Workforce [Internet]. Nih.gov. National Academies Press (US); 2009. Available from: https://www.ncbi.nlm.nih.gov/books/NBK215247/.

28. Heiser S. New Findings Confirm Predictions on Physician Shortage [Internet]. AAMC. 2019. Available from: https://www.aamc.org/news/press-releases/new-findings-confirm-predictions-physician-shortage.

29. Staff. Demand for Specialists Drives Physician Recruitment Shortages [Internet]. www.visionmonday.com. Available from: https://www.visionmonday.com/business/article/demand-for-specialists-drives-physician-recruitment-shortages/.

30. Duquesne University. The Shortage of Healthcare Workers in the U.S. [Internet]. Duquesne University School of Nursing. 2021. Available from: https://onlinenursing.duq.edu/post-master-certificates/shortage-of-healthcare-workers/

31. Rosseter R. Nursing shortage fact sheet [Internet]. American Association of Colleges of Nursing. American Association of Colleges of Nursing; 2022. Available from: https://www.aacnnursing.org/news-data/fact-sheets/nursing-shortage.

32. THE EDITORS. The U.S. Needs More Midwives for Better Maternity Care. Scientific American [Internet]. 2019 Feb; Available from: https://www.scientificamerican.com/article/the-u-s-needs-more-midwives-for-better-maternity-care/.

33. Deakin M. NHS Workforce Shortages and Staff Burnout Are Taking a Toll. BMJ [Internet]. 2022 Apr 11;377(1):945. Available from: https://www.bmj.com/content/377/bmj.o945.

34. Taylor M. Why is there a shortage of doctors in the UK? The Bulletin of the Royal College of Surgeons of England [Internet]. 2020

Mar;102(3):78–81. Available from: https://publishing.rcseng.ac.uk/doi/full/10.1308/rcsbull.2020.78.

35. Chancellor listens to BMA with pension taxation reform to help keep senior doctors in the NHS - BMA media centre - BMA [Internet]. The British Medical Association is the trade union and professional body for doctors in the UK. [cited 2024 Mar 7]. Available from: https://www.bma.org.uk/bma-media-centre/chancellor-listens-to-bma-with-pension-taxation-reform-to-help-keep-senior-doctors-in-the-nhs.

36. Baker C. NHS staff from overseas: statistics. commonslibraryparliamentuk [Internet]. 2022 Nov 22; Available from: https://commonslibrary.parliament.uk/research-briefings/cbp-7783/.

37. McCarey M, Dayan M. Has Brexit affected the UK's medical workforce? [Internet]. The Nuffield Trust. 2022. Available from: https://www.nuffieldtrust.org.uk/news-item/has-brexit-affected-the-uk-s-medical-workforce.

38. Ravikumar S, Thomas N. Workers stage largest strike in history of Britain's health service. Reuters [Internet]. 2023 Feb 6; Available from: https://www.reuters.com/world/uk/britain-faces-largest-ever-healthcare-strikes-pay-disputes-drag-2023-02-05/.

39. NHS England publishes data on junior doctor strike. NHS England [Internet]. 2023 Apr 17; Available from: https://www.england.nhs.uk/2023/04/nhs-england-publishes-data-on-junior-doctor-strike/.

40. You are being redirected... [Internet]. Fraserinstitute.org. 2019. Available from: https://www.fraserinstitute.org/article/canadas-doctor-shortage-will-only-worsen-in-the-coming-decade.

41. Cambridge Dictionary. BUREAUCRACY | meaning in the Cambridge English Dictionary [Internet]. Cambridge.org. 2019. Available from: https://dictionary.cambridge.org/dictionary/english/bureaucracy.

42. Busting bureaucracy: empowering frontline staff by reducing excess bureaucracy in the health and care system in England [Internet]. GOV.UK. 2020. Available from: https://www.gov.uk/government/consultations/reducing-bureaucracy-in-the-health-and-social-care-system-call-for-evidence/outcome/busting-bureaucracy-empowering-frontline-staff-by-reducing-excess-bureaucracy-in-the-health-and-care-system-in-england.

43. NHS still wasting £480m a year on temporary staffing from private agencies, watchdog says [Internet]. The Independent. 2018. Available from: https://www.independent.co.uk/news/health/nhs-agency-locum-doctors-nurses-bank-staff-improvement-spending-a8514871.html.

44. Ford M. NHS agency spend up 20% in England amid workforce gaps [Internet]. Nursing Times. 2022. Available from: https://www.nursingtimes.net/news/workforce/nhs-agency-spend-up-20-in-england-amid-workforce-gaps-14-11-2022/.

45. Wanjiru F. 15 highest-paying countries for doctors in the world in 2021 [Internet]. Tuko.co.ke - Kenya news. 2021 [cited 2024 Mar 7]. Available from: https://www.tuko.co.ke/facts-lifehacks/434208-15-highest-paying-countries-doctors-world-2021/.

46. Davis M. Trainee medics leave university with £100,000 in debt amid cost of living crisis [Internet]. The Mirror. 2023 [cited 2024 Mar 7]. Available from: https://www.mirror.co.uk/news/uk-news/trainee-doctors-leaving-university-over-28956755.

47. Zavlin D, Jubbal KT, Noé JG, Gansbacher B. A comparison of medical education in Germany and the United States: from applying to medical school to the beginnings of residency. GMS German Medical Science [Internet]. 2017 Sep 25;15. Available from: https://www.ncbi.nlm.nih.gov/pmc/articles/PMC5617919/.

48. Winslow CE . A. THE UNTILLED FIELDS OF PUBLIC HEALTH. Science [Internet]. 1920 Jan 9;51(1306):23–33. Available from: https://www.science.org/doi/10.1126/science.51.1306.23.

49. John Hopkins University. Mortality Analyses [Internet]. Johns Hopkins Coronavirus Resource Center. 2023. Available from: https://coronavirus.jhu.edu/data/mortality.

50. Scally G, Jacobson B, Abbasi K. The UK's public health response to covid-19. BMJ [Internet]. 2020 May 15;369. Available from: https://www.bmj.com/content/369/bmj.m1932.

51. Who's who on secret scientific group advising UK government? [Internet]. the Guardian. 2020. Available from: https://www.theguardian.com/world/2020/apr/24/coronavirus-whos-who-on-secret-scientific-group-advising-uk-government-sage.

52. Mahase E. Covid-19: UK advisory panel members are revealed after experts set up new group. BMJ. 2020 May 5;m1831.

53. David Buck [Internet]. 2020. Available from: https://www.kingsfund.org.uk/sites/default/files/2020-01/LGA%20PH%20reforms%20-%20final.pdf.

54. Thomas C. Hitting the poorest worst? How public health cuts have been experienced in England's most deprived communities [Internet]. IPPR. 2019. Available from: https://www.ippr.org/blog/public-health-cuts.

55. Gov.UK. Transforming the public health system: reforming the public health system for the challenges of our times [Internet]. GOV.UK. 2021. Available from: https://www.gov.uk/government/publications/transforming-the-public-health-system/transforming-the-public-health-system-reforming-the-public-health-system-for-the-challenges-of-our-times.

56. Oliver E, Segaren N. More UK doctors should do public health training. BMJ. 2013 Apr 24;f2443.

57. Allan GM, Lexchin J. Physician awareness of diagnostic and nondrug therapeutic costs: A systematic review. International Journal of Technology Assessment in Health Care [Internet]. 2008 Apr 1 [cited 2022 Sep 21];24(2):158–65. Available from: https://www.cambridge.org/core/journals/international-journal-of-technology-assessment-in-health-care/article/abs/physician-awareness-of-diagnostic-and-nondrug-therapeutic-costs-a-systematic-review/DF9E506FAA530AD8D2487D92AEC27D91.

58. Outcomes for graduates (Tomorrow's Doctors) [Internet]. Available from: https://www.gmc-uk.org/-/media/documents/Outcomes_for_graduates_Jul_15_1216.pdf_61408029.pdf.

59. How much money does the NHS waste? BBC News [Internet]. 2016 Oct 21; Available from: https://www.bbc.co.uk/news/health-37715399.

60. Coronavirus: Spending watchdog questions plan to burn unused PPE. BBC News [Internet]. 2022 Jun 10; Available from: https://www.bbc.co.uk/news/uk-politics-61749657.

61. NHS England. The NHS Long Term Plan [Internet]. NHS Long Term Plan. 2019. Available from: https://www.longtermplan.nhs.uk/publication/nhs-long-term-plan/.

62. Norman G, Bennett P, Vardy ERLC. Virtual wards: a rapid evidence synthesis and implications for the care of older people. Age and Ageing [Internet]. 2023 Jan 1;52(1). Available from: https://academic.oup.com/ageing/article/52/1/afac319/6974849?login=false&s=09.

63. Government plans 500% expansion of virtual wards [Internet]. Digital Health. 2023. Available from: https://www.digitalhealth.net/2023/01/government-plans-500-expansion-of-virtual-wards/.

64. Schultz K, Vickery H, Campbell K, Wheeldon M, Barrett-Beck L, Rushbrook E. Implementation of a virtual ward as a response to the COVID-19 pandemic. Australian Health Review. 2021;45(4):433.

65. NHS England. 2022/23 Priorities and Operational Planning Guidance [Internet]. 2022 Feb. Available from: https://www.england.nhs.uk/wp-content/uploads/2022/02/20211223-

B1160-2022-23-priorities-and-operational-planning-guidance-v3.2.pdf.

66. NHS England. NHS Long Term Workforce Plan [Internet]. NHS England. 2023 Jun. Available from: https://www.england.nhs.uk/wp-content/uploads/2023/06/nhs-long-term-workforce-plan-v1.2.pdf.

67.What is the NHS budget. What is the NHS budget? [Internet]. Full Fact. 2019. Available from: https://fullfact.org/health/what-is-the-nhs-budget/.

68.The King's Fund. NHS funding: our position [Internet]. The King's Fund. The King's Fund; 2022. Available from: https://www.kingsfund.org.uk/projects/positions/nhs-funding.

69. Adult Social Care: Key facts And figures [Internet]. The King's Fund. Available from: https://www.kingsfund.org.uk/insight-and-analysis/data-and-charts/key-facts-figures-adult-social-care.

70. NHS England» NHS Operational Planning and Contracting Guidance 2020/21 [Internet]. www.england.nhs.uk. Available from: https://www.england.nhs.uk/publication/nhs-operational-planning-and-contracting-guidance-2020-21/.

71. The rise and decline of the NHS in England 2000-20 [Internet]. Available from: https://assets.kingsfund.org.uk/f/256914/x/0ab966500b/rise_decline_nhs_england_2000-20_2023.pdf.

72. Anandaciva S, Murray R. Reforming the finances of the NHS [Internet]. The King's Fund. 2020. Available from: https://www.kingsfund.org.uk/publications/reforming-finances-NHS.

73. Exploring NHS and Social Care Funding Options [Internet]. www.rand.org. Available from: https://www.rand.org/randeurope/research/projects/nhs-social-care-funding-options.html.

74. Flawed data? Why NHS spending on the independent sector may actually be much more than 7% [Internet]. British Politics and Policy at LSE. 2019 [cited 2024 Mar 7]. Available from: https://blogs.lse.ac.uk/politicsandpolicy/nhs-spending-on-the-independent-sector.

75. How to understand public sector spending [Internet]. GOV.UK. [cited 2024 Mar 7]. Available from: https://www.gov.uk/government/publications/how-to-understand-public-sector-spending/how-to-understand-public-sector-spending.

76. Tikkanen R, Osborn R, Mossialos E, Djordjevic A, Wharton G. Norway | Commonwealth Fund [Internet]. The Commonwealth FUnd. 2020. Available from: https://www.commonwealthfund.org/international-health-policy-center/countries/norway.

77. Healthcare for UK nationals living in Norway [Internet]. GOV.UK. Available from: https://www.gov.uk/guidance/healthcare-in-norway.

78. Healthcare in Norway [Internet]. www.helsenorge.no. 2023 [cited 2024 Mar 7]. Available from: https://www.helsenorge.no/en/healthcare/.

79. Australian Institute of Health and Welfare. Health system overview [Internet]. AIHW. 2022. Available from: https://www.aihw.gov.au/reports/australias-health/health-system-overview.

80. Biggs A, Cook L. Health in Australia: a quick guide - August 2018 update [Internet]. Semantic Scholar. 2018 [cited 2024 Mar 7]. Available from: https://api.semanticscholar.org/CorpusID:216884502.

81. Biggs A. Medicare and health system challenges [Internet]. Parliament of Australia. 2015. Available from: https://www.aph.gov.au/About_Parliament/Parliamentary_Departments/Parliamentary_Library/pubs/BriefingBook45p/MedicareChallenges.

82. Reader E. Do you really need private health insurance? Here's what you need to know before deciding - Easy Reader [Internet]. easyreader.org. [cited 2024 Mar 7]. Available from: https://easyreader.org/article/page/theconversation/do-you-really-need-private-health-insurance-heres-what-you-need-to-know-before-deciding-93661.

83. Parliament of Australia. Health overview [Internet]. www.aph.gov.au. 2022. Available from: https://www.aph.gov.au/About_Parliament/Parliamentary_Departments/Parliamentary_Library/pubs/rp/BudgetReview202223/HealthOverview.

84. Rice T, Rosenau P, Unruh L, Barnes A. Health Systems in Transition United States Health system review. 22:2020. Available from: https://iris.who.int/bitstream/handle/10665/338880/HiT-22-4-2020-eng.pdf?sequence=1.

85. Mar 13, 2019. Most Medicare Beneficiaries Lack Dental Coverage, and Many Go Without Needed Care [Internet]. KFF. [cited 2023 Sep 30]. Available from: https://www.kff.org/medicare/press-release/most-medicare-beneficiaries-lack-dental-coverage-and-many-go-without-needed-care/.

86. Medicaid Managed Care Market Tracker [Internet]. KFF. 2019. Available from: https://www.kff.org/data-collection/medicaid-managed-care-market-tracker/.

87. MAANI N, GALEA S. COVID-19 and Underinvestment in the Health of the US Population. The Milbank Quarterly. 2020 May 13;98(2):239–49.

88. Capitation [Internet]. www.nhis.gov.gh. Available from: https://www.nhis.gov.gh/capitation.aspx.

89. Jacobson G, Damico A, Published TN. Medicare Advantage 2019 Spotlight: First Look [Internet]. KFF. 2018 [cited 2024 Mar 7]. Available from: https://www.kff.org/medicare/issue-brief/medicare-advantage-2019-spotlight-first-look.

90. Rice T, Quentin W, Anell A, Barnes AJ, Rosenau P, Unruh LY, et al. Revisiting out-of-pocket requirements: trends in spending, financial access barriers, and policy in ten high-income countries. BMC Health Services Research. 2018 May 18;18(1).

91. Kane C. Recent Changes in Physician Practice Characteristics [Internet]. 2021 [cited 2024 Mar 7]. Available from: https://www.ama-assn.org/system/files/2021-06/june-2021-ppps-ed-session-slides-carol-kane.pdf.

92. Doty MM, Tikkanen R, Shah A, Schneider EC. Primary Care Physicians' Role In Coordinating Medical And Health-Related Social Needs In Eleven Countries. Health Affairs. 2020 Jan 1;39(1):115–23.

93. Urgent Care Association Industry White Paper – The Essential Role of the Urgent Care Center in Population Health. (Urgent Care Association, Nov. 2019) {Internet}. Available from :https://urgentcareassociation.org/wp-content/uploads/2023-Urgent-Care-Industry-White-Paper.pdf.

94. Fast Facts on US Hospitals [Internet]. Available from: https://www.aha.org/system/files/media/file/2020/01/2020-aha-hospital-fast-facts-new-Jan-2020.pdf.

95. Hartman M, Martin AB, Benson J, Catlin A. National Health Care Spending In 2018: Growth Driven By Accelerations In Medicare And Private Insurance Spending. Health Affairs. 2020 Jan 1;39(1):8–17.

96. Vital and Health Statistics Series 3, Number 43 Vital and Health Statistics [Internet]. 2019. Available from: https://www.cdc.gov/nchs/data/series/sr_03/sr03_43-508.pdf.

97. 2022 Best Practices in Healthcare Survey [Internet]. WTW. Available from: https://www.wtwco.com/en-us/insights/2023/01/2022-best-practices-in-healthcare-survey.

98. Parker R. 60 years of the NHS [Internet]. the Guardian. The Guardian; 2017. Available from: https://www.theguardian.com/society/2008/jun/22/nhs60.nhs1.

99. NHS Hospital Bed Numbers: Past, Present, Future [Internet]. The King's Fund. Available from: https://www.kingsfund.org.uk/insight-and-analysis/long-reads/nhs-hospital-bed-numbers.

100. Worldometers. U.K. Population (2023) - Worldometers [Internet]. Worldometers. 2023. Available from: https://www.worldometers.info/world-population/uk-population/.

101. HM Revenue & Customs. Percentile points from 1 to 99 for total income before and after tax [Internet]. GOV.UK. 2012. Available from: https://www.gov.uk/government/statistics/percentile-points-from-1-to-99-for-total-income-before-and-after-tax.

102. Billionaire Charlie Munger Labels US Healthcare A "Disgrace" as Report Shows Lowest Life Expectancy Despite Highest Spending [Internet]. Yahoo Finance. 2023 [cited 2024 Mar 7]. Available from: https://finance.yahoo.com/news/billionaire-charlie-munger-labels-us-183520169.html?fr=sycsrp_catchall.

103. Developing countries can respond to COVID-19 in ways that are swift, at scale, and successful [Internet]. Brookings. Available from: https://www.brookings.edu/articles/developing-countries-can-respond-to-covid-19-in-ways-that-are-swift-at-scale-and-successful/.

104. Nsofor IM, Mormina M. What developing countries can teach rich countries about how to respond to a pandemic [Internet]. The Conversation. 2020. Available from: https://theconversation.com/what-developing-countries-can-teach-rich-countries-about-how-to-respond-to-a-pandemic-146784.

105. African Union rolls out Partnership to Accelerate COVID-19 Testing | African Union [Internet]. au.int. [cited 2024 Mar 7].

Available from: https://au.int/en/pressreleases/20200603/african-union-rolls-out-partnership-accelerate-covid-19-testing.

106. Commission Decision C(2014) 2258 final [Internet]. health.ec.europa.eu. Available from: https://health.ec.europa.eu/publications/commission-decision-c2014-2258-final_en.

107. Taylor L. Uruguay is winning against covid-19. This is how. BMJ. 2020 Sep 18;m3575.

108. Mutesa L. Rwanda's COVID-19 pool testing: a savvy option where there's low viral prevalence [Internet]. The Conversation. 2020 [cited 2024 Mar 7]. Available from: https://theconversation.com/rwandas-covid-19-pool-testing-a-savvy-option-where-theres-low-viral-prevalence-141704.

109. Win T.L, Peyton, N, and Mataishe F. With drones and masks, African innovators keep COVID-hit economies afloat. Reuters {Internet}. July 7, 20207:25 AM GMT; Available from : https://www.reuters.com/article/idUSKBN2480O7/.

110. Jones L, Palumbo D, Brown D. Coronavirus: How the pandemic has changed the world economy. BBC News [Internet]. 2021 Jan 24; Available from: https://www.bbc.co.uk/news/business-51706225.

111. Gould CC. Transnational Solidarities. Journal of Social Philosophy. 2007 Mar;38(1):148–64.

112. Meredith S. Rich countries are refusing to waive the rights on Covid vaccines as global cases hit record levels [Internet]. CNBC.

2021. Available from: https://www.cnbc.com/2021/04/22/covid-rich-countries-are-refusing-to-waive-ip-rights-on-vaccines.html.

113. Should the UK Government use technology to transition from the COVID-19 public health crisis? [Internet]. www.adalovelaceinstitute.org. Available from: https://www.adalovelaceinstitute.org/news/exit-through-the-app-store-uk-technology-transition-covid-19-crisis/.

114. Doctors and nurses worldwide point to roadmap to future-proof healthcare | Elsevier [Internet]. www.elsevier.com. [cited 2024 Mar 7]. Available from: https://www.elsevier.com/about/press-releases/doctors-and-nurses-worldwide-point-to-roadmap-to-future-proof-healthcare.

www.ingramcontent.com/pod-product-compliance
Lightning Source LLC
Chambersburg PA
CBHW070305230526

45470CB00002B/727